Surviving HIV/AIDS in the Inner City

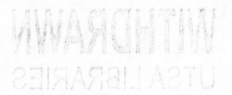

Surviving HIV/AIDS
in the Inner City

How Resourceful Latinas
Beat the Odds

SABRINA MARIE CHASE

RUTGERS UNIVERSITY PRESS

NEW BRUNSWICK, NEW JERSEY, AND LONDON

LIBRARY OF CONGRESS CATALOGING-IN-PUBLICATION DATA

Chase, Sabrina Marie.
  Surviving HIV/AIDS in the inner city : how resourceful Latinas beat the odds /
Sabrina Marie Chase.
      p. ; cm. — (Studies in medical anthropology)
  Includes bibliographical references and index.
  ISBN 978-0-8135-4892-0 (hardcover : alk. paper) — ISBN 978-0-8135-4937-8
(pbk. : alk. paper)

  1. HIV-positive women—New Jersey—Newark—Case studies.   2. AIDS (Disease) in
women—New Jersey—Newark—Case studies.   3. Puerto Rican women—Diseases—
New Jersey—Newark—Case studies.   I. Title.   II. Series: Studies in medical
anthropology.
  [DNLM: 1. HIV Infections—ethnology—New Jersey.   2. HIV Infections—psychology—
New Jersey.   3. Healthcare Disparities—New Jersey.   4. Hispanic Americans—
psychology—New Jersey.   5. Urban Health Services—New Jersey.   6. Women's
Health—ethnology—New Jersey.   WC 503.7 C487s 2011]
  RA643.84.N49C43   2011
  362.196′979200974932—dc22   2010013762

A British Cataloging-in-Publication record for this book is available
from the British Library.

Manufactured in the United States of America

For Nini

CONTENTS

LIST OF FIGURES AND TABLES

Figures

Tables

ACKNOWLEDGMENTS

The resourceful women of Newark, Elizabeth, and New Brunswick, New Jersey, made this book possible through the generous gifts of their time, trust, and friendship. Both they and their families took a chance by taking me under their wings. Many others also deserve thanks for this book and I cannot hope to name them all. Charles Jones, Providencia Gavilanes, Ana Santiago, Ellen Abdunafi, Michelle Chatman, Pushpinder Pelia, "Cuqui" Rivera, Laharry Pittman, Karen Sorrell, River Huston, and Geane Chatman all offered me kindness, support, inspiration, and insight just when I needed it.

Numerous social service agencies welcomed me. The staff of each went out of their way to include me in workshops and other activities. I'd like to thank, in particular, the New Jersey Women and AIDS Network (NJWAN), the Union County HIV Consortium Resource Center, CURA, Hyacinth, the St. Columba Neighborhood Club, the Puerto Rican Action Board, the Red Ribbon Fellowship, PROCEED, and Us and Them. I am grateful, also, to the doctors, nurses, and staff of the clinics and health care offices that allowed me to accompany women on their health care appointments.

Without the support of a National Institute of Mental Health (NIMH) Minority Dissertation Research grant, the fieldwork that produced this book would never have happened. The Rutgers Institute for Health, Health Care Policy, and Aging Research offered me a graduate fellowship when I left the field and the Research Division of the Department of Family Medicine at UMDNJ–Robert Wood Johnson Medical School accepted me into their National Research Service Award (NRSA) Health Services Research Postdoctoral Fellowship program. Both fellowships allowed me to analyze my data and write successively better drafts of the manuscript. Igda Martinez, Denise Davis, and Joann Donatiello at the Rutgers Center for State Health Policy provided unstinting help and support at a critical time in the writing process. Sarah Avery-Davis moved mountains and braved terrible memories from her own dissertation process to make sure that I finished on time.

Many teachers and scholars invested in me to bring this project to fruition: Peter Guarnaccia, Louisa Schein, Caridad Souza, and Ana Ramos-Zayas read multiple drafts and offered numerous wonderful suggestions. Dr. Schein and

Dr. Guarnaccia in particular offered unstinting intellectual and emotional support throughout many years of work. Catie Willging and Lisa Vanderlinden gave me the practical support I needed to keep the project moving forward. Later on, Sandra Echeverría gave me hope and helped me reframe a number of key concepts. This book would never have been completed without her support. Hanaa Hamdi offered encouragement and helped me find a way to assist the Newark AIDS community. The wise, perceptive comments of Michele Tracy Berger and Nancy Romero-Daza provided me with direction when I wasn't sure where to go. Of course, all errors and oversights that remain are my own.

Cat Castells, Tracy Colatarci, and Stéphanie Thill read endless chapters and suggested numerous improvements. Keith Campbell created a beautiful mock book cover for me to post on my wall for inspiration and chose the final photo. Oliver Lontok collaborated with my husband, Michael Brown, to help me triumph over the vagaries of EndNote and format the text. The tables and graphs that so poignantly show the impact of cultural and social capital on the lives of Newark's women are the brainchild of Cat Castells, who also worked hard to keep me sane during end-stage revision. My husband, Michael Brown, created the final versions of these tables and figures, making them exceptionally beautiful. Brooke Goode served both as a mentor and copyeditor, gently guiding me through the latter stages of the revision process. Coop and Syndy Smith contributed their time and energy to the project, helping to move me forward with the semifinal set of revisions. Barbara DiCicco-Bloom worked hard to preserve my work time and provided emotional support for well over a year. She and Rebecca Etz read excerpts of the manuscript and offered practical feedback. Finally, Dr. Benjamin Crabtree offered intellectual, emotional, and pragmatic support. His wise advice got me off the treadmill of endless revisions, and his vision for the future of health care reminded me why I do this every day. Likewise, John Scott and Jeanne Ferrante helped move this manuscript forward and gave me a clearer understanding of what great primary and specialty care might look like. Of course, I am forever grateful for the inspiring work of Paul Farmer, Margaret Connors, Merrill Singer, Nancy Scheper-Hughes, Jay Macleod, Philippe Bourgois, and Emily Martin.

These acknowledgments would never be complete without thanking my family and friends, who loved and supported me throughout the endless writing process. My husband and life partner, Michael Brown, inspires me more than I can say and makes every day worth living. My parents, Charles and Cida Chase, gave me everything I needed to become a balanced, healthy person capable of this work. They've also encouraged me to think carefully and choose wisely whenever great choices are to be made. I am thankful for their love and guidance. My brother, Christopher W. Chase, has been a loving source of encouragement and support over the many years it took me to finish this project. Finally, I am thankful to the many as-yet unmentioned friends who never allowed me to lose sight of what is most important: Karen Abbott, Lisa Curran-Slatterback, Jennifer Hamilton, Dan Davis, Dorothy Weaver, Phyllis Fry, Meagan Cummings, Barbara Dove, Beth Somerville, Bill Metrey, Linda Julian, George Marvil, Katie Birckmayer, Patrick Fagan, Kayla Serotte, Lori Sinatra, Peter Flister, Renee Cyr, Bill Seligman, Mathew Callahan, the entire Smith-Rowland family (Peggy, Ed, Rose, Audrey, and Ben), Shannon Bowman, Martha Smith, Steve Robinson, Jennie Rodigue, Tom Murphy, Wendy Birky, and the entire Blue Star community. Thank you, now and always.

ABBREVIATIONS

AA	Alcoholics Anonymous
ADAP	AIDS Drug Assistance Program
AIDS	Acquired Immunodeficiency Syndrome
ARC	AIDS-Related Complex
AZT	Azidothymidine
CAM	Complementary and alternative medicine
CBO	Community-based organization
CDC	Centers for Disease Control and Prevention
DYFS	Division of Youth and Family Services
GMHC	Gay Men's Health Crisis
GRID	Gay-related immune deficiency
HAART	Highly Active Anti-Retroviral Therapy
HERS	HIV Epidemiology Research Study
HIV	Human immunodeficiency virus
HOPWA	Housing Opportunities for Persons with AIDS
HUD	U.S. Department of Housing and Urban Development
ID clinic	Infectious disease clinic
IDU	Injection drug user
IVDU	Intravenous injection drug user
JAMA	*Journal of the American Medical Association*
MSM	Men who have sex with men
NA	Narcotics Anonymous
NJWAN	New Jersey Women and AIDS Network
OI	Opportunistic infection
PCP	Pneumocystis carinii pneumonia
PWA	Person with AIDS
RARE	Rapid assessment, response, and evaluation
SAVA	Substance abuse, violence, and AIDS
SIDA	Síndromo de Immunodeficencia Adquirida (Spanish acronym for AIDS)
SRO	Single-occupancy hotel room

SSDI   Social Security Disability Insurance
SSI   Supplemental Security Income
UMDNJ   University of Medicine and Dentistry of New Jersey
WIHS   Women's Interagency HIV Study

Surviving HIV/AIDS in the Inner City

1

Torn between Structure
and Agency

"Anywhere the struggle is great, the level of ingenuity and inventiveness is high."

—Eleni Gabre-Madhin

Caridad and her son, Manuelito, had lived in Newark for only a year when she got married. This was an unexpected blessing. Caridad had left Puerto Rico to escape an abusive relationship with her longtime partner, a violent IV drug user. When she arrived she hoped only for a peaceful life; she had not expected to fall in love again so soon. Her new husband, Eduardo, was an older man, who had also been born in Puerto Rico. It had been a whirlwind courtship—some said too brief—but Caridad was bursting with happiness and hope. They shared common values: like her, he was religiously observant and never used drugs. Eduardo was also completely accepting of her HIV-positive status. When Caridad explained that she had contracted the virus from her previous partner, he told her that he was not afraid—he wanted to embrace everything about her. After their marriage, the three of them settled into a small apartment and began living life as a family.

A few months later, Caridad began experiencing abdominal pain, cramping, and vaginal bleeding. Her symptoms first appeared on a weekend, so she and Eduardo went to the emergency room at Mercy Hospital in Newark. Had it been a weekday, she would have used Mercy's Marshall Clinic, the closest thing she had to a primary care doctor. But the clinic was closed on weekends, so Caridad went to the emergency room at Mercy instead. She hoped that if she was lucky, she might be able to see one of the doctors who worked at her clinic.

When she arrived and explained her symptoms to the triage nurse, she and her husband were separated from the other ER patients. They waited a long time—not uncommon—but Caridad spent the time wondering if they had been put in isolation because of her HIV-positive status. When she finally saw a doctor, he examined her, performed some tests, and told her that she was pregnant.

Unfortunately, he added, she was also in the middle of a miscarriage. She would need a D&C (dilation and curettage—a procedure in which the cervix is expanded so the uterine lining can be scraped away) immediately. Caridad was shocked and distressed. Her religious convictions made abortion impossible. She knew she did not want a D&C if there was any chance that the baby would survive. But if the baby was already dead, she would accept it. Caridad tried to explain this to the doctor, asking him if he was sure that the baby was already dead. But he became impatient with her resistance. When she pressed him, refusing to make a decision without an absolute assurance, he snapped, "Why are you so worried about it? You are HIV-positive—you had no business getting pregnant anyway!" With that, he left the room, leaving the two of them to piece together their options and decide what to do. They had no money for a second opinion, so they decided to go home and call the Marshall Clinic on Monday to ask for an emergency appointment. This meant waiting for a day and a half while Caridad continued to bleed. It also meant grappling with stress, discomfort, and fear. But after the emergency room doctor's rejection, she felt she had no better options.

Mondays at the Marshall Clinic are always packed because everyone who misses a Thursday or Friday appointment calls on the following Monday. Luckily, Caridad got an appointment, but her husband had just started a new job and could not go with her. She was anxious about going alone, so she called me. We waited for hours in the crowded anteroom as Caridad worried about the bleeding and what to do about her son. He would be released from his daycare at 4 P.M. Someone had to pick him up and that someone could not be late. The child of any parent who was over twenty minutes late would be dropped from the center. Caridad had worked hard to get Manuelito's daycare placement, which freed her to attend a computer/secretarial training class so she could find a job. Without the daycare, she would lose this opportunity.

Because the family could not afford a car, Eduardo would have had to leave early to pick up Manuelito, so he could not go. Caridad couldn't even reach him by phone. As a security guard, he stopped near a phone only once an hour. As we waited, I called Caridad's friends, looking for someone who could pick up Manuelito and keep him for a few hours if necessary. Caridad hoped to see a doctor early enough to get her son on time, but as we waited, this seemed less and less likely.

By early afternoon Caridad was desperate. A motherly African American woman with a kind face noticed her distress and asked what was wrong. As Caridad's story spilled out, the lady listened intently, patting my friend's thigh in a comforting way. Finally, Caridad asked the woman what she thought we should do. In a low voice, the lady suggested an entirely new strategy. Why not leave the clinic now, use the bus to pick up her son, and then go to the emergency room at Trinity Hospital? Once there, Caridad should say nothing about her affiliation with the Marshall Clinic. Instead, she should present herself as an emergency case who had seen no one today. Our advisor reasoned that once we had Manuelito, we could bring him with us and I could watch him in the ER waiting room while Caridad saw a doctor. Additionally, Trinity was widely known for its friendly staff and good care. Perhaps Caridad might find a sympathetic ear. And, said our new friend, emergency cases were seen quickly at Trinity. But Caridad could not admit that she was a regular patient at the Marshall Clinic. If she did, they would probably just send her back here.

I could see that Caridad was thinking through her options. If she left immediately, she would still be bleeding, but she would reach her son before four o'clock. But if she stayed and sent me to pick him up, she might face a painful decision alone. The quality of care at Trinity was also important; Caridad had heard good reports about the Trinity emergency room. I had also seen evidence that they offered excellent care when I accompanied our mutual friend Nini to the emergency room there less than a year before.

While Caridad struggled, I made another phone call, this time to Nini. Miraculously, she answered. She agreed to hop on the bus and pick up Manuelito, saying she could keep him overnight if necessary. Relieved that he was in good hands, we were about to leave for Trinity when the triage nurse appeared. She had reordered the afternoon patient charts, putting Caridad at the head of the line. The doctor treated Caridad gently and with great care. He examined her closely, asking questions, and listening carefully. After noting her condition in the chart, he told us that Caridad needed to be admitted to the hospital immediately. Without missing a beat, he called in the nurse and asked her to take us to a lower floor where Caridad would receive a sonogram that might be able to determine what had happened to the baby.

Downstairs, I held Caridad's hand while they administered the test. Another doctor pored over the results for a long time and then called me aside. Quietly, she told me that she thought the fetus was dead, but she could not be absolutely 100 percent sure. However, she was certain that Caridad needed to be admitted immediately. The doctor's compassion was obvious as she urged me to talk my friend into staying so they could schedule a D&C.

When I explained this to Caridad, she became even more frightened. She desperately wanted to talk to Eduardo, saying she couldn't check into the hospital without him. Could she go and find him, and come back later? Gently, the physician explained that if Caridad left the hospital, there would be another long wait when she returned. They could not hold a hospital room for her. They couldn't even schedule a procedure if she walked out now. I watched the doctor during the exchange: she looked worried, though she spoke very calmly. Her tone was urgent. Softly, I tried to talk Caridad into checking in by herself while I took the bus to find Eduardo. Torn and wavering, Caridad stood in the hall and wept. The nurses whispered to each other and glanced at us nervously as we stood in a little circle of privacy.

Finally, Caridad decided that she needed to share the decision with her husband. I tried to negotiate with the staff: was there any way to avoid the wait when we came back? Could we see one of the doctors who already knew about Caridad's case? After some thought, the physician told us that she would be on another floor of the hospital if we didn't return too late. She told us to ask the emergency room receptionist to go and get her as soon as we arrived and she would help if she could.

This was more than I expected. With a heavy heart I followed Caridad out of the hospital. We walk to the bus station, waited, and transferred to another bus before reaching Eduardo. As we traveled, Caridad cried and I searched my backpack for enough change to take a taxi. There was none to be found. An hour later we got off the bus and I spotted an ATM. After a quick stop there, we found Eduardo. He got permission to leave early and we all climbed into the taxi that took us back to the hospital. The receptionist found the doctor who had helped Caridad, and within minutes, she and Eduardo consulted the physician together. In the end, the couple decided that they would proceed with the D&C. I left them alone in a hospital room holding hands and whispering.

Caridad's story, taken from a field note written in 1999, offers us a glimpse of the structural violence faced by poor HIV-positive women living in the United States. Structural violence can be thought of as hardships that result from "neither nature nor pure individual will . . . but . . . historically given (and often economically driven) processes and forces that conspire to constrain individual agency" (Farmer, Simmons, and Connors 1996). For many women living in U.S. urban settings, structural violence appears in the form of poverty, lack of resources, AIDS-related stigma, and the synergistic combination known as SAVA: substance abuse, violence, and AIDS (Singer 1994; Singer 1996). Caridad's story offers us a glimpse of her confrontation with each in turn. In it, we can see how they endangered her health, her life, and her family, while invoking tremendous stress and fear.

But the story doesn't end there. It also suggests that women like Caridad and her waiting room mentor—poor HIV-positive women of color—can draw on their intelligence, experience, and social networks, acting as effective agents on their own behalf. At great personal risk, Caridad succeeded in getting the care she needed on her own terms with the assistance of key allies. She demanded and got additional information about the health of her fetus. She drew on a reservoir of data about the resources available. She held out for a joint decision with her husband. She upheld her most important values about the sanctity of life, even in the face of one doctor's contempt. If we attend to the whole picture of poor urban women's experience without underestimating either their agency or the power of the structural violence they face, we can learn a great deal about success and failure in the face of overwhelming odds. This book is about poor HIV-positive Puerto Rican women like Caridad. But it is not about how to enhance HIV/AIDS prevention or how to eliminate structural violence. There are scores of other excellent books and articles about these critically important topics. This book is about how women deal with the structural violence they cannot change, and what this can teach us about supporting them, and each other, more effectively.

Caridad belonged to a small group of HIV-positive Latinas who allowed me into their lives from 1997 to 2000. About half of these women had never used intravenous (IV) drugs. They had contracted the virus from husbands or long-term partners with a history of injection drug use. The others acquired HIV either from IV drug use or drug-related sex work. All seventeen women spent most of their time taking care of their children, grandchildren, and men. If they had any energy left over, they took care of themselves. None had private insurance or enough money to pay their bills every month. Each woman depended on some form of government support to make ends meet.

Caridad and her cohort all identified themselves as Puerto Rican, though some used the term "Boricua," while others preferred "Spanish." Seven had been born in New York or New Jersey, while ten had been raised in Puerto Rico and moved to the greater Newark area as adults or teens. They all loved Newark's diverse, Spanish-speaking community, embracing the vibrant city as their home. Its challenges were as familiar to them as its delights.

Many of the women in my study were accustomed to the poverty, unemployment, and drug problems that hounded their neighborhoods, but each was shocked to discover that she was HIV-positive, despite the fact that New Jersey was on the leading edge of the nation's HIV/AIDS epidemic. The state had first reported the nation's highest proportion of HIV-positive women in 1984, when they accounted for 15 percent of the state's 443 known AIDS cases (Leusner 1990a).

By June of 1990, women made up 21 percent of New Jersey's AIDS cases (Leusner 1990a). Over half of them had contracted HIV through intravenous drug use and the rest had acquired the disease from sexual relations with an infected male partner. Half of these women didn't know their partner was using drugs or putting them at risk (Leusner 1990b). When the *Journal of the American Medical Association* (*JAMA*) reported that AIDS was the leading killer of black women of child-bearing age in New York and New Jersey, 1,159 New Jersey women had already died (Chu, Buehler, and Berkelman 1990; Leusner 1990a). Almost all the women I worked with knew at least one person who had died of AIDS at the time of their own diagnosis in the early-to-mid 1990s, but that person was usually a man. Despite Newark's longstanding HIV epidemic, few women in my study imagined that they could be at risk.

Here, you will find the stories and lessons they shared with me. I was surprised to learn that women who could "cross" into ethnic and social groups other than their own used this familiarity to great advantage. They befriended doctors, advocates, social workers, nurses, home health care workers, and other valuable allies with relative ease. Because of this, they were given more time, attention, information, and resources than other equally needy and equally deserving women. Looking through the lens of social science theory, these women had a broad "cultural- and social-capital toolkit."

It wasn't simply that some women were friendlier or more charming than others. I met a number of very charming, friendly women who consistently struggled with feelings of social awkwardness, insecurity, and even hostility when faced with unfamiliar environments, institutions, and gatekeepers. During my fieldwork, I observed that they struggled to advocate for themselves in both health care and social service settings. They had to work harder to recruit and retain helpers and allies. But women who were already comfortable with the social norms and behavioral expectations of white, black, and Latino middle-class workers were well positioned to turn almost any gatekeeper—anyone who controlled access to a resource—into an ally.

These experienced women arrived at their diagnosis with track records of successful interaction with bureaucratic systems dominated by middle-class workers. Once diagnosed, they used skills honed much earlier to extract more than the typical amount of help from clinic, agency, and hospital staff. The most successful women in my study—those able to find "extra" resources for themselves and others—could tap the expertise of poor and working-class allies as well.

But they were the exception, not the rule. Most of the women who worked with me were like the rest of us: comfortable with the unspoken rules that run our communities and disoriented when forced outside of them. The majority of the women I worked with were much more effective at operating inside of their own familiar *habitus*, or "class, and subculture-specific worldview" (Bourdieu 1986).

In the everyday world, it might be awkward to try to guess the unspoken rules governing a new environment: "What are those little muslin nets covering the lemons at this fancy restaurant, and what do I do with them? Will the waiters laugh if I fumble with them?" But in hospitals, clinics, and social service agencies, the stakes are much higher. In these settings, chronically ill women (and men) who "fumble" risk alienating important potential allies—doctors, nurses, and social workers. They may miss out on critical information. They can face ongoing indifference or even hostility as a result. When resources are scarce, as they are in poor inner-city settings, losing allies can have severe long-term consequences.

While these lessons tell us something about the subtle aspects of health care disparities, they are also relevant for anyone managing a chronic disease or serious medical condition. Those who understand the nuances of our health care delivery system and the preferences of the people who run them will receive better care—and often experience better outcomes—than those who do not. My observations suggest that our urban health care system, in particular, delivers high quality care mostly to those best equipped to extract it.

This book asks four sets of questions about the women in my study: Given their limited resources, how did they manage an illness as serious as HIV/AIDS? Did they seek out alternatives to conventional medical treatments, and if so, what kind? Did the magnitude of the challenges they faced deprive them of agency, or could they act effectively on their own behalf and that of others? If so, how did their agency operate? And what can we, as a greater society, learn from this? What can Newark's resourceful women teach us about our health care system and the way we can expect to use it?

The Help-Seeking Pathways Study

In the broadest sense, my study touched the lives of a large group of Puerto Rican, black, and white HIV-positive women, their husbands, children, physicians, nurses, therapists, alternative health care professionals, social workers, agency workers, neighbors, friends, and clergy. I encountered this larger group in clinic waiting rooms, agency functions, conferences, churches, and other HIV/AIDS community gatherings. Over time, they grew to know me and my work. Many were generous with their help and eager to share their insights, and some specifically asked to be included in some way. But the great bulk of my study focused on a small group of seventeen HIV-positive Puerto Rican women who allowed me intimate access to their lives. I followed them through their daily routines for about three years, interviewing them repeatedly over the course of my fieldwork.

The women in this group were wholly or partially dependent on the public health care system. None had private health insurance. Some had Medicaid, the nation's medical insurance program for those living below the poverty level. A few had both Medicaid and Medicare, its counterpart for seniors and people living with one of several designated disabilities. A few had no insurance at all. Most women were between thirty and thirty-nine years of age, three were older and one was younger. Ten were born in Puerto Rico and moved to the United States in their youth; seven were born on the mainland. All traveled back and forth to the island regularly. At least eleven women acquired HIV from a husband or long-term boyfriend. Almost half of these believed their partners had given them the virus knowingly, while choosing to keep their HIV status a secret.

Only two women were completely open about their HIV-positive status. Thirteen disclosed it exclusively in the private and semipublic spaces of their local HIV/AIDS community, or the socially integrated group of people, spaces, and activities organized around HIV-related services, activism, and treatment. While all thirteen women participated in HIV/AIDS community activities, they kept this a secret from neighbors and even some family members. Two women were almost completely closeted. They shared their HIV status only with clinicians, social workers, and one or two others. These two women did not consider themselves part of the wider HIV/AIDS community. They entered my study only because they had a close friend or ally who was already participating.

When I began planning my research in 1995, New Jersey ranked fifth in the nation for total number of individuals living with AIDS, and third for the number of women and children infected with HIV. At that time, New Jersey had more adult and adolescent females with AIDS per hundred thousand people than any other state (New Jersey Department of Health 1994). Most of these cases (and most documented cases of HIV) were clustered within Essex County, although there were a large number of cases in Middlesex County as well.

For this reason, I chose to focus on three field sites: Newark and Elizabeth (both in Essex County) and New Brunswick (in Middlesex County). All but three of the women I worked with lived within the largest Metropolitan Statistical Area (MSA) in northern New Jersey, the Newark MSA. An MSA is a geographic region encompassing a large central city and its outlying areas; it is often thought of as an extended city (Acosta-Belén and Santiago 2006, 136). I spent most of my time in three infectious disease clinics, one in each city. I also worked with four hospitals, seven social service agencies, and in the homes and neighborhoods of the women I followed. HIV-related conferences, lectures, agency fund-raisers, workshops, peer education initiatives, and support groups provided a greater context for this study.

In this cautious community, snowball sampling was a useful way to locate and enroll study participants. This technique, especially useful for working with hard-to-reach and "hidden" populations, works through the power of referrals. Once a "cultural expert" has been recruited, she or he works with the researcher to introduce the project to other eligible individuals (Bernard 1994). With the help of Nini, a knowledgeable and well-respected HIV/AIDS-community member, I was able to overcome the secrecy so many used to shield themselves from HIV's powerful stigma. Patience was required to gain the community's trust, but Nini vouched for my character, discretion, and trustworthiness and asserted the value of my study to her HIV-positive peers, doctors, community workers, support group leaders, allies, and even clinic directors. Through Nini, I was introduced to HIV-positive Puerto Rican women who connected me to others in turn.

Once I began field research in 1998, I engaged in participant observation, conducted unstructured and semistructured interviews, and accompanied women to their health care appointments (Bernard 1994). I collected observational data from diverse groups of HIV-positive women and men, health care practitioners, social workers, agency and clinic staff, women's health activists, peer counselors, HIV-test specialists, researchers, and HIV/AIDS activists, many of whom became my friends. During the course of my research, I audiotaped semi-structured interviews, open-ended conversations, various lectures, and two medical consultations. I spoke both Spanish and English, allowing the women I accompanied to choose the language they preferred. Most of the time, we spoke "Spanglish," since almost everyone was comfortable using a mix of the two languages; only three women preferred Spanish, and only one preferred English.

In planning and executing this study, I followed the guidelines of the Rutgers University Institutional Review Board (IRB). Because HIV/AIDS is a highly stigmatizing condition that can lead to social ostracism, I obtained informed consent through the use of verbal consent scripts. This was done to avoid creating a paper trail recording participants' HIV status. Outside of the HIV/AIDS community, I explained that I was studying Puerto Rican women's use of the health care system, avoiding any disclosure of women's HIV status. Finally, in writing this book, I have altered details of women's appearance, household structure, and other identifying characteristics in order to protect their confidentiality.

As part of my work, I offered reciprocity whenever possible. My guides gave me their time and attention. They shared their thoughts and concerns, allowing me into their therapeutic consultations and private lives. In return, I tried to offer them things of value. At the most basic level, I gave out (very) modest payments. Every few visits, I gave each participant twenty dollars until they had received one hundred dollars. In the cases of a few women who were more difficult to reach, I gave it out in two or three larger sums.

While this was useful, it was only the beginning. As I became more familiar with each woman's life, I began to look for things I could do that might make her days easier. Most women were fairly quick to point out what I could do to help them. Since few could afford a car, they traveled by bus or sometimes by taxi, and I was often asked to help carry heavy bags. On the days we traveled together I would haul bags of groceries, household goods, and sometimes cases of Ensure (a liquid calorie and vitamin supplement). In the same spirit, I sometimes helped transport massive bags of laundry and fold clothes.

I also gave each woman my undivided attention, listening to her thoughts and dreams and lessening periods of loneliness and isolation. I acted as a translator, typed up and sent out formal letters, and accompanied women to family or divorce court when needed. I especially enjoyed advocating for women when asked to do so. I was frequently asked to help obtain medical files and remind women to ask particular questions during consultations. Sometimes women turned to me for help remembering what had happened during previous visits, and at times, I vouched for women operating under stress, explaining the challenges they faced to impatient and overwhelmed doctors, nurses, and social workers.

Quickly, I found myself drawn into women's help-seeking strategies. For example, Celestina asked me to remind each doctor, nurse, and assistant we encountered who I was and what I was doing whenever I accompanied her. She pushed me to do this even when it became repetitious because she thought her clinicians would be much more thorough under my watchful eye. Eventually, I came to agree with her.

However, our system of reciprocity went well beyond my original expectations. When my role as a poor graduate student left me broke, Nini and Nerina sent me home with food from their own pantries. Celestina, Nini, and Deborah regularly gave me generous portions of chicken with arroz con gandules (rice with pigeon peas) so I wouldn't have to cook dinner for my husband after my long commute home. When Nini redecorated her kitchen, she gave me two sets of matching curtains and hand towels. On days in which Gabrielle, Selma, Nini, Celestina, or Nerina suspected that I was angry or sad, they would urge me to talk and they would listen for a little while. In this way, my work brought me deeply into the lives of my friends, guides, and informants, and embedded them just as deeply into my own. Over time, I slowly began to understand the many challenges they faced.

Before HIV: Poverty, Prejudice, and Health Disparities

Even before discovering their HIV-positive status, the women in my study grappled with poverty, inequality, and prejudice. The literature on Puerto Rican poverty often describes Puerto Ricans as the most economically and socially disadvantaged group of Northeastern Latinos (Perez 1994; Cruz 2003; Elmelech and Lu 2004; López 2007). Puerto Rican families living on the U.S. mainland have lower incomes, higher poverty and unemployment rates, and greater numbers of female-headed households than either Mexicans or Cubans, the other two largest U.S. Latino groups (Baker 2002; Acosta-Belén and Santiago 2006). And although they are citizens, Puerto Rican citizenship has not been treated as equal to that of other U.S. citizens. Instead, "Puerto Ricans have been politically and economically treated as second-class with minimum representation in matters concerning their fate" (Baker 2002, 49). Finally, the poverty and prejudice faced by Puerto Rican women is compounded by gender-related disadvantages, putting them at the mercy of "intersectional stigma," or a complex assortment of inter-related biases, the sum of which is greater than its individual parts (Berger 2004).

Even when compared to other disadvantaged groups, such as African Americans and other Latinos, Puerto Ricans earn notably lower incomes (Baker 2002; Acosta-Belén and Santiago 2006). In the South, of the various racial and ethnic groups, non-Hispanic whites had the highest mean family income in one 1990–1995 study sample, followed by Cubans and Mexicans. African Americans trailed behind all three, but Puerto Ricans had by far the lowest family incomes of all groups examined (South, Crowder, and Chavez 2005, 884). Looking at this from a slightly different perspective, the 1990 mean income of Puerto Ricans was only 59 percent of the U.S. average, and by 2000, this figure had climbed to only 61 percent (Acosta-Belén and Santiago 2006, 111). Educational attainment is closely linked to income, so it is important to note that mainland Puerto Rican communities struggle with high rates of high school dropout and low rates of bachelor and postgraduate education. Regionally, communities in the Midwest and Northeast (where Puerto Rican populations are highest) struggle the most, with a 55.6 percent dropout rate in the former and a 53.5 percent dropout rate in the latter (Baker 2002, 84).

The persistent, long-term nature of Puerto Rican poverty has generated a great deal of debate, but the situation can be summed up in a way on which most researchers and social policy advocates can probably agree.

> What was said about poverty and politics in Puerto Rico in 1949 could be said today about Puerto Rican poverty and politics on the mainland: the promise of participation and access to power remains unfulfilled. Despite some measure of upward mobility, the overall socioeconomic status of Puerto Ricans remains low; moreover, they seem unable to follow in the path of those groups to whom politics was kinder. Worse yet, American social and economic systems have failed Puerto Ricans. (Cruz 2003, 154)

On the mainland, most Puerto Ricans live in Northeast and Midwest urban centers like New York, Philadelphia, Chicago, Newark, and Hartford, where they are often segregated into very poor neighborhoods (Acosta-Belén and Santiago 2006). The concentration of Puerto Ricans in troubled Northeastern cities can be described as "pockets of extreme poverty surrounded by an infrastructure in decline" (Acosta-Belén and Santiago 2006, 143). To make matters worse, Puerto Ricans stand out among other disadvantaged groups as having unusually low probabilities of escaping them. Only 5.4 percent of Puerto Ricans moved from a high-poverty neighborhood to a lower poverty neighborhood, as compared to 8.5 percent of Mexicans, 9.1 percent of Cubans, 10.6 percent of non-Latino Blacks, and 17.3 percent of non-Latino whites in one study (South, Crowder, and Chavez 2005, 882). This results from a web of factors: most Puerto Ricans are born into poorer neighborhoods, they are more likely than whites to rent rather than own their own homes, and, unlike home owners, they are more likely to move to higher poverty areas (South, Crowder, and Chavez 2005, 896). This implies that Puerto Ricans are also less likely than other groups to escape poverty itself—not just poorer neighborhoods.

When the health of mainland Puerto Ricans is compared with that of other Latino groups, significant differences emerge. Cubans and Mexicans, for example, enjoy better health than Puerto Ricans, and in general, Puerto Ricans have a more negative health profile and a clearer pattern of health disparities than other major groups (Hajet, Lucas, and Kingston 2000; Zsembik and Fennell 2005, 57). The effect of culture on health also varies among Latino subgroups, and Spanish-language preference may play a more significant role for Puerto

Ricans than for other Latinos. Spanish-speaking Puerto Ricans have more medical conditions than English-speaking Puerto Ricans, and Puerto Rican immigrants, too, have more medical conditions and functional impairments than those born on the mainland. For other Latinos, language preference appears to have a less striking impact on disparities (Zsembik and Fennell 2005). Finally, the relationship of socioeconomic status to health outcomes also varies among Latino subgroups. For Puerto Ricans, income appears to be the most critical factor to adversely affect health, but for Mexicans, education and insurance coverage appear to matter the most (Zsembik and Fennell 2005).

While citizenship has not put Puerto Ricans on the same footing as other, more advantaged citizen groups, it has given Puerto Rican men and women better access to health insurance than other Latinos. In a comparison of Mexican, Cuban, and Puerto Rican women, Puerto Ricans had the highest rate of health insurance coverage (de la Torre et al. 1996, 536). As citizens, they had access to publicly subsidized health insurance programs like Medicaid, the nation's state-administered health care program for poor women and men. Citizenship facilitates access to state and federal programs not only because citizens can meet program eligibility requirements more easily, but because they do not have to fear revealing an undocumented status in order to access care.

Despite this advantage, the women in my study faced significant challenges. Their gender added to the biases they faced. Minority women in general tend to be younger, less educated, more likely to live in poverty, and less likely to have access to health care than their male counterparts. Their educational attainment rates are lower, they often lack a regular source of care, and as minority group members, they wrestle with inaccessible health care, language barriers, and lack of culturally sensitive care (Glanz et al. 2003; Elmelech and Lu 2004). However, Puerto Rican women fare even worse than many of their minority group counterparts.

When comparing male and female poverty rates among Puerto Ricans, whites, blacks, Asians, Mexicans, Central/South Americans, and American Indians, the greatest income inequality emerges between Puerto Rican men and women. For men, a study noted a poverty rate of 17.6 percent, while for women it was a stunning 32.4 percent, representing one-third of all Puerto Rican women—the highest poverty rate for females of any group. This gap of nearly 15 percent exceeded that found among all other groups. Only the 10.7 percent gender poverty gap between black men and women could even approach it (Elmelech and Lu 2004, 165).

SAVA: An Urban Syndemic

The women who worked with me faced these challenges from within troubled urban communities. They and their neighbors lived at or below the poverty level, jobs and childcare were scarce, local schools were poorly funded, and illegal drugs were ubiquitous. Most had friends and relatives who grappled with addictions of one kind or another, and I was surprised that so many told me of family members who had died of AIDS. In short, they had a great deal in common with other inner-city residents, especially those living in New York, Philadelphia, Baltimore, Hartford, and Washington, D.C. Even the residents of Midwestern cities like Detroit and Chicago wrestled with similar problems (Berger 2004; Chambré 2006; Bowser, Quimby, and Singer 2007; Bergmann 2008).

The Centers for Disease Control and Prevention (CDC) tell us that 85 percent of the United States' cumulative AIDS cases have been reported in large metropolitan areas (Kaiser 2007). The cities of the Northeast have consistently reported the highest AIDS case rates. More recently, there were 21.1 cases of AIDS reported per 100,000 people in this region as a whole as of 2005, compared to 16.9 in the South, 8.9 in the West, and 7.4 in the Midwest. New York currently reports the highest number of AIDS cases, New Jersey ranks fifth, Pennsylvania sixth, and Maryland ninth (CDC 2009). Most of these occur in urban communities of color. In 2006, nearly half of all new diagnoses (49 percent) occurred among blacks, 18 percent among Latinos, and only 30 percent among whites (CDC 2009).

The urban nature of HIV/AIDS in the United States has not gone unnoticed. Medical anthropologist Merrill Singer argues that any discussion of HIV/AIDS must be firmly anchored in its inner-city context, acknowledging "a broader set of political economic and social factors, including high rates of unemployment, poverty, homelessness and residential overcrowding, substandard nutrition, environmental toxins and related environmental health risks, infrastructural deterioration and loss of quality housing stock, forced geographic mobility, family breakup and disruption of social support networks, youth gang and drug related violence, and health care inequality" (Singer 1994, 933).

Further, he notes that this environment of deprivation and suffering makes inner-city communities especially vulnerable to drug traffickers, who can offer both jobs and a source of temporary escape. When jobs and opportunities are scarce, these are attractive lures. But substance abuse creates an increased risk of exposure to HIV and other sexually transmitted diseases (STDs), which can become cofactors in HIV infection. Intravenous drug use is especially dangerous, greatly increasing the likelihood that intravenous drug users (IVDUs) will contract the virus through needle sharing and then transmit it to others via sex, new needle-sharing partners, and/or pregnancy (Singer 1994).

Inner-city women are at greater risk than their suburban counterparts whether they inject drugs or not, because they are more likely to encounter sexual and romantic partners with a history of injection drug use. They are also more likely to both witness and experience violence and sexual abuse, further elevating their risk (Connors 1996; Romero-Daza, Weeks, and Singer 2005; Frye et al.

2007). In 2006, 80 percent of all U.S. women diagnosed as HIV-positive contracted the virus from high-risk sexual contact (CDC 2009).

Anthropologists Paul Farmer and Margaret Connors have written extensively about poor urban women's enhanced vulnerability to HIV/AIDS. Farmer points out that they are often forced to assent to unprotected sex even when they know their lives are in danger, and young women, in particular, are frequently unable to refuse risky sex (Farmer, Simmons, and Connors 1996, 46). Connors summarizes their precarious position in this way: "For poor women, sex can become a strategy for economic and psychological survival both in cases where sex is engaged in purely for money and drugs, and in relationships where women must depend on their partners for food and rent money" (Connors 1996, 116). Because accessible jobs that pay a living wage are so scarce in inner-city communities of color, enforced economic dependency on men (who may themselves depend on the economic benefits of drug trafficking) is difficult to break. Further, when women do hold sole economic responsibility for a household and children, they are likely to plunge deeper and deeper into poverty, creating an endless cycle of risk (Connors 1996, 53).

Singer names this synergistic blend of substance abuse, violence and AIDS the SAVA "syndemic," arguing that they are mutually reinforcing problems rather than independent dangers: "Diseases do not tend to spread in a social vacuum nor solely within the bodies of those they inflict; thus their transmission and impact are never merely biological. Ultimately, social factors like poverty, racism, sexism, ostracism, stigmatization, disruption of social systems, and structural violence may be of far greater importance than the nature of pathogens or the bodily systems they infect in the transition of the development of epidemics" (Singer and Weeks 2005, 163). But the picture is even more complex. Although the SAVA syndemic can be found in city after city, Singer and others point out that HIV/AIDS isn't really a single, unitary phenomenon at all (Singer 1994; Singer 1996; Baer, Singer, and Susser 1997). Instead, it is an assortment of "multiple, separate micro-epidemics in any given region of our country. Each of these micro-epidemics has its own population, and its own motivators that inform behavior" (Goosby 2007, viii). In essence, SAVA takes root in cities across the nation, unfolding differently in each one. It even varies across neighborhoods of the same city.

As many social scientists and advocates have pointed out, conditions of oppression fuel HIV/AIDS wherever poverty and inequality concentrate. Farmer and Connors are well known for emphasizing the similarities between poor urban women in the United States and rest of the world. All of these women face elevated risks of HIV infection because their lives are remarkably similar. They face the same kind of structural violence: low social status compounded by economic and gender inequality. Given this fact, Connors asserts that the job of the social scientist is to address those structures that place women at great and unequal risk, rather than exaggerating the agency—or independent ability to act—of women with HIV infection (Connors 1996). Here, she is speaking critically of HIV-prevention research that urges women to do exactly the kinds of things that prove almost impossible in the context of SAVA, like negotiating for condom use with men on whom they depend for food and shelter.

Connors is right, and so are Farmer and Singer. Structural violence is exceptionally powerful. It is flourishes in both U.S. and Third World urban centers, and it puts poor women, especially poor women of color, at greater risk while limiting their ability to act as independent agents on their own behalf. But is this the whole picture? Is there anything more to understand?

Theoretical Tools: Using Lenses to Understand the World

If we are to understand what we see on the streets, if we are to make sense of the forces that act upon these [individuals], and if we are to generalize from their experiences in any meaningful way, we must situate our work in a broader theoretical framework by letting theory inform our data, and ultimately, by allowing our data to inform theory. (MacLeod 1995, 10)

Legions of students, readers, and even policy makers have muttered the following questions as they struggled angrily through dense theoretical discussion of serious social problems. Why is theory so important, and why must social scientists frame every discussion of the world's problems with pages and pages of jargon-laden theory? Why can't we simply focus on solving the problems themselves? These are not frivolous questions, and social scientists should not dismiss them or take the answers for granted.

Theories are like lenses through which we see the world. They highlight certain parts of our environment while deemphasizing others. Through each of our theoretical lenses, we can see some aspects of a problem, but no single lens can show us everything that might be important. Theories, like microscope lenses, focus on different levels: some are good for observing macro-level or community-level forces. Others focus on the individual, and tell us something about interpersonal reality. Like microscope lenses, theories are more useful when they arrive in groups. In this way, we can use them together to combine the insights generated by different theories, producing a more complete picture of the problem at hand.

Researchers like Farmer, Connors, and Singer give us crucially important lenses through which to understand structural violence and its impact on individual agency. In the case of HIV/AIDS, their lenses are particularly good for showing us the tremendous risks and barriers that poor urban women of color must face. When we combine their theories with others that have the potential to tell us more about individual agency under conditions of structural constraint, new and important insights can emerge.

The tension between *structure* (the greater social, economic, and cultural forces that shape our lives) and *agency* (the ability to make autonomous choices and act effectively on behalf of ourselves and our communities) is always present when theorizing about oppressed groups and communities. Very few social scientists would deny that poor urban women of color face serious limitations over which they have little control. However, this does not necessarily mean that they are powerless. Social scientists must negotiate the two extremes of portraying them as passive victims and exaggerating the agency they possess. This is notoriously difficult to do.

The problem can be described from a different perspective as confusing subordination with subservience the following way, "To claim that women are not subservient is to demonstrate that they are active subjects and not passive objects. To claim that women are not subordinate is to demonstrate that in all spheres . . . women are not lacking in authority, power and control relative to men" (Oakley 1989, 5). As Ann Oakley notes here, the line between the two is sometimes blurred in anthropological discussions of gender (Oakley 1989, 7). In exploring the stories of Newark's resourceful women, it is important to avoid either trap in order to faithfully represent how victimization and agency can coexist for them in complex, multidimensional ways (Miller 1993; Romero-Daza, Weeks, and Singer 2003). Following sociologist Jay MacLeod and cultural anthropologist Philippe Bourgois, I will use the theoretical lenses of French sociologist Pierre Bourdieu to represent each woman's agency as faithfully as possible without minimizing the structural violence that has shaped her life.

In their own ethnographic analyses, MacLeod and Bourgois each turn to Bourdieu to answer questions about how agency operates within structurally constrained environments, and why some can perform better in the worlds outside of their neighborhoods than others (MacLeod 1995; Bourgois 2003). Taken together, the concepts of *cultural capital, social capital,* and *habitus* can help illuminate the challenges faced by intelligent, resourceful individuals who find themselves helpless when confronted by unfamiliar middle-class institutions, government offices, and bureaucratic agencies. They can also help explain why some poor HIV-positive women of color might function well under these circumstances while others become overwhelmed and give up in the face of so many challenges.

All the women who worked with me confronted structural violence, but some were able to shape their lives in ways that others could not. Despite being buffeted by larger economic, historical, and political forces, Nini, Caridad, Julia, Selma, Gabrielle, Celestina, Nerina, and Deborah usually landed on their feet. They consistently found the best doctors accessible to them and received better care than many of their peers, enjoying longer consultations, commanding greater attention, and getting more than the usual dose of help for their problems. Paquita, Flor, Nilsa, Amelia, Cristina, Juana, and Carlotta, on the other hand, experienced briefer consultations and more cursory care, even when others tried to send help their way. While they were able to build some relationships with doctors and social workers, these relationships were less intense, fewer in number, and less likely to produce resources and benefits improving their lives. Each of these groups has something to teach us about enacting agency in the context of structural violence. They also have unexpected lessons to teach about the way our health care system is structured to both give and deny care.

Contextualizing what I saw in the lives of these women with the work of Farmer, Bourdieu, MacLeod, and Bourgois, I slowly began to make sense of these lessons. Bourdieu's concepts of *cultural capital, habitus,* and *social capital* proved to be especially important in this process (Bourdieu 1986). Bourdieu used the term *cultural capital* to describe a group of important resources that individuals acquire from the families who raise them and socialize them into adulthood. These resources include benefits that spring from the family's cultural background, social class, and legacies of achievement in education, business, or the military. Examples of the latter might include mentorship and guidance from parents and grandparents who had earned advanced degrees, served as military officers or who ran their own businesses. None of these benefits are tangible in the usual sense, but each can bolster success by making it easier for an individual to do well in a particular kind of social setting. Because resources like these are usually transmitted from one generation to another, they tend to channel children into the same social class as their parents. However, some individuals may be exposed to and absorb the cultural capital of different social classes and different ethnic groups if they interact with them early and often enough.

Each group's cultural capital is ultimately expressed as its *habitus* (Bourdieu 1983). This is a class- and subculture-specific worldview that prizes one set of preferences and activities over others. One's *habitus* will emphasize some tastes over others—country music instead of opera, for example. It will highlight the advantages of certain kinds of knowledge rather than others (perhaps valuing master carpentry skills more than technical writing) and it will promote particular behaviors (like early parenting as opposed to summer world travel). Each of the preferences, skill sets, and behaviors that make up the *habitus* will make perfect sense from an insider's point of view. It will convey important cultural capital that helps group members thrive in their own subcultural contexts. At the most basic level, no group's *habitus* is better than any other's: each values what it most needs to know to succeed in its own social and cultural niche.

Because it is so group-specific, cultural capital (and the *habitus* it generates) provides individuals with very specific social toolkits that mark them as members of some groups and outliers of others. These toolkits are apparent whenever individuals speak, act, or otherwise "perform" in public. Bourdieu calls this *embodied cultural capital* (Bourdieu 1983). In this way, cultural capital shapes people such that they can step easily into specific sociocultural roles in ways that feel "natural" and appear effortless. But in reality, the smooth fit between individuals and their socioeconomic class, or between individual actors and their social roles, only seem easy because long infusions of cultural capital have shaped each to the other. A dairy farmer in the Midwest, for example, will acquire the cultural capital that makes perfect sense of her world; she will move through her day with practiced ease. The same is true for her counterpart study-ing political science on the East Coast. But if you switch one for the other, they will both be lost: neither will have the skills, knowledge, or social grammar to function well.

But cultural capital and *habitus* don't tell the whole story. Bourdieu's notion of *social capital*, another crucial resource, is also important. The term social capital describes the kinds of benefits that emerge from relationships built on trust and reciprocity. It refers to the aid and support that people sharing the same social network offer each other (Bourdieu 1986). Social capital can emerge from any trusting relationship, but it is especially relevant in social interactions that include gatekeepers, or people who have the power to grant or deny others access to valuable information and resources. The more diverse the network, the more different kinds of resources can be derived from it. Networks that include individuals of high social or political status or great social power can give their allies special access to important knowledge, expertise, or material benefits. For example, a chef whose close friend runs a law firm has a better-than-average chance of landing a catering contract there; an intern being mentored by a well-known surgeon has an edge in applying to top residencies.

This means that people who can access the *habitus*, or cultural capital, of the most powerful social classes have the potential to tap into greater social capital than those who do not. By virtue of their ability to incorporate individuals with more highly valued resources into their social networks, such persons can gain access to a wide range of important benefits. They can accrue resources more easily and more successfully than those who have been taught only the cultural capital of the working and marginal classes.

It is important to understand that this does *not* mean that middle- or upper-class cultural capital is better than the cultural capital of the impover-ished or working classes. Each group treasures and teaches the knowledge that its members depend on the most. Therefore, each *habitus*—each kind of cultural capital—is equally crucial in its own native context. Expertise in portfolio management probably won't help a woman living below the poverty line in rural Georgia, and ten years of making delicious homemade jams won't help a Harvard law student, either. Each needs the kind of knowledge that will help her thrive in the particular place she lives. However, a *habitus* associated with the middle or upper class will allow its hosts greater access to political and economic power, because these social classes control most of our country's formal institutions and economic resources. This suggests that institutions like hospitals and clinics will be most accessible to those whose *habitus* has been shaped by middle- and upper-class privilege, and they will be least responsive to people whose *habitus* has equipped them to function best in impoverished or working-class settings.

This was certainly true in the public hospitals and federally funded clinics where the women I worked with received their care. They depended on the collaborative alliances they forged—their social capital—almost every day. For them, the partnerships they built with health care professionals, administrators, and case managers could literally mean the difference between life and death (Bourdieu 1986). Those who were comfortable with only their own *habitus* struggled to connect with the multiethnic middle- and upper-class professionals around them. Those who preferred Spanish rather than English found themselves at a distinct disadvantage, since most gatekeepers were native speakers of English. But this factor alone did not determine whether a woman would create dependable relationships with resources managers. Some who preferred Spanish (like Celestina and Caridad) forged and maintained many key bonds, while others who spoke fluent English (like Amelia and Nilsa) solidified only a few. Only women who had a broad familiarity with more than one *habitus*—especially that of white middle- and upper-class professionals—were almost always able to recruit gatekeepers from any background into their social networks.

Women with an average toolkit of cultural and social capital, who preferred to stay within their own native *habitus*, found the road much more difficult. Their struggles paralleled those of the African American and Latino men who worked with MacLeod and Bourgois. For these men, failure to negotiate new behaviors in an unfamiliar *habitus* resulted in underemployment, lack of job security, job loss, frustration, and depression. Even when they recognized the "gaps" in their cultural capital and attempted to bridge them, they usually found themselves at a loss. Unsure of what was happening and unable to discern what they should do next to settle into the worlds of middle-class gatekeepers, they found themselves uncomprehending, anxious, angry, or paralyzed, like many of the women with whom I worked. And as Bourgois notes, the result of repeated frustrated attempts to bridge these gaps was often a retreat into the limiting but familiar structural constraints of their home communities of color (Bourgois 2003). For the women in my study, it often meant a retreat back into their own homes, families, or neighborhoods, away from the resources of clinics and social service agencies.

Few would disagree that our current medical system is significantly flawed. Research has demonstrated the existence of a wide range of racial and ethnic disparities in health and health care (Fiscella et al. 2000; Smedley, Stith, and

Nelson 2003). People whose class or culture situates them outside of the white middle class are most at risk of receiving inferior care. No matter what measurement criteria are used, their health outcomes lag behind those of their more privileged counterparts (Smedley, Stith, and Nelson 2003). This is true even when individual clinicians work hard to offer everyone care of the highest quality. Income, geographic location, and insurance status help shape these problems. But they seem even more daunting through the lens of mismatched cultural and social capital, which exacerbates existing disparities. Though we may try to fix the system through modest structural changes and cultural competency workshops, more will be required. Biases born from conflicting cultural capital are subtle, deep, and hard to pin down, as the experiences of Paquita, Flor, Nilsa, Amelia, Cristina, Juana, and Carlotta can attest.

These challenges are daunting, but we should not turn away from them. Paquita deserved the same quality of care enjoyed by Nini. She did not get it, and because of this her life was shorter and sadder than it could have been. No one's story should end this way. Designing a system that provides high-quality health care for everyone is among the most critical problems we must solve today.

This book is an exploration of many things: how urban Latinas survive HIV, what they can teach us about health care disparities, and how New Jersey's heterosexual HIV/AIDS epidemic foreshadowed the country's from the start. These women's stories focus our attention on the urban health care system, challenging us to explore parts of it that desperately need fixing. They paint a picture of intelligent, resourceful women who can be thwarted, but not necessarily defeated. Although structural violence is powerful, it does not always divest individuals of their agency. Complex issues like these are more likely to command our attention when they are embodied in the stories of people whose suffering we can imagine in our own lives, and I am grateful to the women and men who allowed me into their worlds so I could learn these lessons. It is my hope that these stories will make Newark's resourceful women more visible and at the same time promote change in our ailing health care system. This was certainly the hope of the women who shared their lives with me.

2

Resourceful Women

Here you will meet New Jersey's resourceful women through my eyes. I tell these stories with the full awareness that I have, in some sense, constructed them. Though I have drawn from women's own words whenever possible, they do not speak for themselves. If they did, they might say something else. Still, I weave together what I believe to be key elements of their stories, with special attention to their use of cultural and social capital.

I did not understand the power of crossing social and cultural boundaries with ease when I began this project. As a medical anthropologist, it was a daily struggle to cross from my world into the world of Newark's resourceful women. I constantly encountered strange new words, attitudes, and behaviors that left me puzzled, confused, and anxious. Walking down Newark's streets, I felt alone and out of place. Watching young men who should have been healthy use canes to cross the street shocked me, and my friends' constant struggles depressed me. But I took comfort in the knowledge that anthropologists often experience fear and anxiety when they enter an unfamiliar cultural setting (see Berger's 2004 study of HIV-positive women in Detroit for a particularly fitting description of this phenomenon). This distress is often called "culture shock," and it is a normal experience for anyone acclimating to a new environment. Another way to think about culture shock is to say that this is what happens when someone wanders outside of a safe and familiar *habitus.*

I began my study by accompanying each woman to her health care appointments instead of collecting life histories or analyzing social networks. I also administered two audiotaped, semistructured interview guides to each woman, usually in her own home. In these interviews, I asked about the range of medical and mental health care professionals women used, paying special attention to any complementary and alternative practitioners they consulted. I also asked about home remedies and why they had chosen them. Over time, I watched and listened as women sought help from a variety of sources, taking notes in blank books and fleshing them out each night at home. Taped interviews were transcribed and downloaded into a qualitative data management program called NUDIST and coded for emergent themes. Field notes were often typed and then coded and analyzed by hand. Gradually, as I spent time with each woman, I began to learn her story. Over multiple meetings and numerous tellings, the shape of her history began to appear. Such tellings were always partial, and sometimes they shifted over time. Michele Berger describes this kind of emergent process and the analysis that accompanies it from her study of HIV-positive activists, advocates, and helpers in Detroit:

> I argue that one creates oral narratives from people's "raw" data. I have shaped, studied, and coaxed meanings from the data. It has my stamp of authorship on it. What I have collected over the past few years are in the category of oral narratives; they are not technically life stories, they are not solely semistructured interviews, nor are they typical oral histories. They are narratives, sometimes, vignettes, or episodes picked over and worked on, sifted through time and awareness, reattuned for precise moments by respondents and myself. (Berger 2004, 79)

Like Berger, I have used quotes and excerpts from my field notes, sifting through them to offer a snapshot of what I saw. I have combined them with quotes taken from coded interview transcriptions to create a brief glimpse of each woman's life and the way in which she discovered and dealt with her own diagnosis.

Most of the women I worked with spoke a combination of Spanish and English, switching frequently from one language to the other. To make reading easier, I have translated most of their Spanish words and phrases into English. I kept the original Spanish and added a translation in brackets when it was especially important to preserve the original meaning. Caridad, Celestina, Carlotta, and Juana preferred Spanish over English, and their words have been translated whenever they appear, with small exceptions. All translations were reviewed by at least two native speakers of Spanish, one Puerto Rican and one Costa Rican.

I entered the field thinking that I knew at least some of the right questions to ask and understood something about what was important. In retrospect, I was wrong most of the time. Thankfully, each woman directed me to what she thought was most important, gently guiding me away from my questions and into her own.

Although they shared the challenges of an urban HIV-positive life, these women were very different from each other (See Tables 2.1 and 2.2). A tremendous amount of ethnographic and qualitative research has been conducted by anthropologists, sociologists, and other social scientists dedicated to understanding

TABLE 2.1
Women by Cultural-Capital Category

	Birthplace	Age	Education	Religion
Broad capital				
Caridad	Puerto Rico	28	Some college/technical school	Catholic
Celestina	Puerto Rico	37	Some college/technical school	Catholic
Deborah	United States	38	Some college/technical school	Catholic amd New Age
Gabrielle	Puerto Rico	51	Didn't finish high school	Santeria
Julia	Puerto Rico	51	Didn't finish high school	Santeria and New Age
Nerina	United States	51	Didn't finish high school	Santeria and New Age
Nini	United States	39	Some college/technical school	Santeria amd herbalism
Selma	United States	31	Some college/technical school	Not religious
In the middle				
Alicia	United States	34	Didn't finish high school	Not religious
Luchita	Puerto Rico	34	Didn't finish high school	Pentecostal
Average capital				
Amelia	United States	38	Didn't finish high school	Not religious
Carlotta	Puerto Rico	39	Some college/technical school	New Age Spirituality
Cristina	United States	32	Didn't finish high school	Not religious
Flor	Puerto Rico	39	Didn't finish high school	Not religious
Juana	Puerto Rico	37	Didn't finish high school	Jehovah's Witness
Nilsa	Puerto Rico	39	Didn't finish high school	Pentecostal
Paquita	Puerto Rico	39	Didn't finish high school	Evangelical Christian

TABLE 2.2

Risk Factors for HIV

	Substance abuse	Reported sexual abuse	History of sex work	Reported domestic violence or threats of violence	Believed acquired from a partner	Believed acquired from IV drug use
Broad capital						
Caridad	N	Y	N	Y	Y	N
Celestina	N	N	N	N	Y	N
Deborah	Y	Y	Y	Y	N	?
Gabrielle	Y	Y	Y	Y	N	Y
Julia	Y	?	?	?	?	?
Nerina	Y	Y	Y	Y	N	Y
Nini	N	N	N	Y	Y	N
Selma	Y	Y	N	Y	Y	N
In the middle						
Alicia	N	N	N	N	Y	N
Luchita	N	N	N	N	Y	N
Average capital						
Amelia	N	N	N	N	Y	N
Carlotta	N	N	N	N	Y	N
Cristina	Y	Y	Y	Y	?	?
Flor	Y	N	N	N	Y	N
Juana	N	N	N	N	Y	N
Nilsa	N	N	N	Y	Y	N
Paquita	N	N	N	N	Y	N

and ultimately eradicating HIV (for more about this as well as a few sample studies, see Singer and Weeks 1996; Singer, Scott et al. 2001; Singer, Simmons et al. 2001; Weeks et al. 2001; Heimer et al. 2002; Needle et al. 2003; Kim, Peragallo, and DeForge 2006; Heimer et al. 2007). This research often focuses on active and former drug users, their networks, and related high-risk activities like sex work and injection drug use. Some studies seek to understand how women grapple with addiction, risk of HIV/AIDS, and sex work in unforgiving urban environments (Romero-Daza, Weeks, and Singer 2003; Romero-Daza,

Weeks, and Singer 2005), while others emphasize the meanings and agency that HIV-positive women construct from their experience (Berger 2004; Siegel, Schrimshaw, and Lekas 2006). This study falls primarily into the latter tradition, although it seeks to draw on insights from the former. While everyone I worked with was profoundly impacted by someone's drug use, two-thirds had little or no direct experience with drugs or sex work themselves. The attitudes and experiences of these women differed considerably from those of their drug-experienced counterparts. In this respect, my sample and my study differs from most others. Although both groups of women faced similar challenges, they disagreed on many topics. It was very common for women who had never used drugs to voice suspicion and resentment of those who had.

The women in my study split along religious lines as well. Some were Catholic, and would never consider having an abortion, while others felt that it was wrong to give birth to a child who might contract the virus. A few belonged to more evangelical Pentecostal-style churches: these women disapproved of those who practiced Santeria, a Caribbean religious tradition combining African and Catholic belief systems. Consequently, I learned to be very, very careful when answering one woman's questions about another—even when they were good friends. The Pentecostal women I worked with also differed dramatically from each other. One was almost completely closeted, because her pastor condemned HIV-positive people, saying that they were sinners. The other was an openly HIV-positive youth minister whose nontraditional, activist pastor had brought HIV/AIDS education into their church.

Initially, I noticed that everyone in this diverse group depended on collaborative alliances with health care professionals, social workers, and program administrators. In other words, they attempted to use their social capital to solve daily problems. Over time, I noticed that those who had mastered only one *habitus* had a more difficult time commanding and keeping the attention of these professionals. They had to work harder to get less help. But women who moved across one *habitus* after another found it much easier to get assistance. One way to think about it is to imagine a continuum with the most successful self-advocates at one end, and those who struggled the most at the other. Women fell all along the continuum, but most fell closer to either one end or its opposite.

Nini, Julia, Deborah, Nerina, Selma, Celestina, Gabrielle, and Caridad (see Table 2.1) fell closer to the flexible end of the continuum. They moved between various social classes and ethnic groups with relative ease. Most had acquaintances and friends of multiple ethnicities and backgrounds. Cristina, Nilsa, Carlotta, Flor, Paquita, Juana, and Amelia all fell closer to the less flexible end of the continuum. They showed the average person's hesitance when crossing ethnic and class-related boundaries. Each of these women knew her native *habitus* well, but showed considerable discomfort outside of it.

Luchita and Alicia landed somewhere in the middle. They forged one or two key alliances outside their native *habitus* and cultivated them heavily. For example, Luchita's outspoken, HIV-savvy pastor brought her into the church's social network and monitored her physician's treatment decisions. Alicia developed a close relationship with a well-known local HIV/AIDS activist from the African American community who connected her to a good doctor, an HIV resource center, and others like herself.

Broad Cultural and Social Capital: Nini, Caridad, Julia, Deborah, Celestina, Nerina, Selma, and Gabrielle

Nini

Nini was born and raised in Newark. As a preteen, she lived with relatives in Puerto Rico, returning to the city of her birth at the age of twenty. When we met at the annual New Jersey Women and AIDS conference in Newark, Nini was about to turn forty.

We began chatting while applying makeup in front of a bathroom mirror at the conference hotel. When I explained who I was and described my research, she generously invited me to visit her, saying she'd be happy to show me how to get around the city and maneuver through the HIV-positive world. We exchanged phone numbers and agreed to talk. But when I searched for it later, the number was gone; I was left only with the memory of a vivacious woman who had offered me guidance.

The following year I returned with funding and a stack of bright purple flyers introducing my study in Spanish and English. I made plans to meet the first person to call my toll-free number. As I walked toward the McDonald's at Newark Penn Station, a strangely familiar woman waited for me, and I saw my flash of recognition mirrored in her own. It was none other than Nini, the woman from the hotel bathroom, who would become my friend and primary teacher over the next three years.

Nini explained that shortly after her second marriage, she had been diagnosed with cancer. While in recovery from the operation to treat it, she heard some stray hospital gossip about a woman who had just tested HIV-positive. Later, she learned that this story was about her. "I had an operation . . . a tumor . . . and as part of it, they gave me a test. Afterward, [my doctor] told me . . . You better believe it was a shock. I've only had sex with two people, and it was my husband who gave it to me. Then I found out he already knew about it. I hit him with a chair when I found out."

The physician who coordinated her cancer care also spent several days a week working at one of the largest infectious disease (ID) clinics in the

Northeast. Because of this coincidence, Nini entered an ID clinic right away under the care of her own doctor. He had been born and trained among the upper classes of Central America, while she had grown up in modest neighborhoods in Newark and Puerto Rico. Yet her middle-class work history and community college training brought their worlds a little closer. Nini also shared his distaste of drug use, which solidified their bond. And though Dr. Sergio had thousands of patients to care for, he developed a special interest in helping her, even giving her his pager number.

> I am lucky, and I know it. Dr. Sergio gave me his pager number. Other patients don't. . . . I know he treats me better than he treats other patients. . . . If I hadn't gone to Dr. Sergio for my stomach bleeding seven months ago, I would have died. I went to the ER at Mercy and they said it was nothing much. But I didn't believe them. I went to see Dr. Sergio and he did the tests and found the bleeding. . . . He said, "You know that if anything happens you've got the beeper number." None of his patients at the clinic have the beeper number. I have his office number and his mailbox, too. He told me, "If I have to meet you, I'll meet you." He knows I will not sell drugs or call him if it's not serious. The bleeding was a good example of this. I would have died without him.

After her diagnosis, Nini fought anger and depression for some time. "I flipped out when I found out," she told me. "I mean, I really flipped out." But she also found herself with a strange advantage compared to others at the clinic. She knew everyone who was anyone, and she also knew how to transform acquaintances into allies. After activating her contacts and doing a little informal questioning, she knew every social service agency in the greater Newark area and what each of them had to offer. Soon she knew something about HIV services at each specialty clinic and metropolitan hospital in the city as well. She used this knowledge to decide where to go in conjunction with her clinicians.

NINI: I don't feel good. I'm having trouble breathing. Monday I am going to the hospital.

SABRINA: What hospital? Why?

NINI: I went to the coo-coo doctor [her psychiatrist] and asked to be put in the hospital. I'm going to Trinity, not Mercy. I don't feel like myself.

Nini had a wide repertoire of interactive styles, or what Pierre Bourdieu calls "embodied cultural capital" (1986). She was familiar with the biases and expectations of both the middle and working classes and used this knowledge to her benefit. For example, Nini noticed that the clinic personnel were uncomfortable with boisterous conversation. And though she loved to talk and laugh loudly among her neighborhood friends, she was careful to lower her voice around clinicians. Nini was also hyperaware that middle-class professionals often assumed that HIV-positive women were either drug addicts or prostitutes. This infuriated her, but it also informed her behavior. She took great pains to let everyone in the clinic know that she had never taken drugs or slept around; she dressed and spoke in a conservative manner that distanced her from drug use and signaled respectability.

Previous exposure had taught Nini how to work with bureaucratic systems and extract what she needed. Her familiarity with Newark's many ethnic enclaves also meant she was comfortable in most settings. This helped caregivers and professionals of many backgrounds feel comfortable around her, making it that much easier for them to help. In this way, her flexibility in crossing from one *habitus* to another worked to her advantage. She used this advantage to help others in Newark's HIV/AIDS community cultivate similar strategies, with various degrees of success.

Caridad

Through Nini, I met Caridad, a vibrant twenty-eight-year-old woman born in Puerto Rico. Caridad had lived in Newark for less than a year when we met. She told me that she had been tested for HIV in Puerto Rico during her first semester of college. When she confronted her boyfriend with the positive test result, he confessed to injecting drugs. Caridad was seventeen at the time. She decided to stay with him, but he soon began to hit her, steal her money, and sell her possessions to buy drugs. Several years after the birth of their son, a friend invited her to move to Newark, and Caridad was able to escape.

> I came on September 10. And on October 11, I will never forget it, [my friend] threw me out in the street because her husband robbed me. Then I told her and she said no, that I had to go, that he had not robbed me. Then since he was such a manipulator, she believed him. She told me, "Look for everything because you are leaving." And I left. I sat down there across the street with my bags and the baby. . . . I left for a church, down there, a church by a basement. There I was about a month, in that church, with a mattress like this. Like this was the mattress. The mattress was so thin, on the floor, with the baby. It was very cold. They did not approve the welfare, I had no one to help me, I did not know English, imagine.
>
> Well, I met some friends from Puerto Rico; they gave me dishes and things like that. Afterward I went to work; I took care of some babies in the basement. There at the church I got some babies to care for from the people that went there to church, who were Methodist. I worked eighteen hours a day, for four months, in order to pay for a basement. Then I moved

to another basement, to a room, with the baby. The gentleman from there gave me a bed, a little table; a friend gave me a little table, another one gave me another little table.

By extending and rebuilding her social network, Caridad generated the resources to move into a new apartment. However, she soon discovered that her former boyfriend had followed her to Newark and was asking where she could be found. Ever resourceful, she lay low until he gave up and left. Despite her difficulties, she was determined to begin a new life. Her only regret was that she had not finished her college education. She had been most interested in pharmacy, but had enjoyed the whole experience.

I studied a little bit at the university. At the university it was a requirement to study biology, metaphysics, physics, and that is interesting. That is
the study of the human being; it is very important because the mind is the
most powerful thing that you have. If you think that a finger is hurting,
and continue to think my finger is hurting, this finger is hurting, and [if]
you forget that that finger is hurting, you can be sure that you will forget
that finger. Then [if] you are [thinking]: "Oh if I am sick, and oh this is
bothering me, and oh this is destroying me." If you think like that then you
are truly going to destroy yourself. You don't have to think like that.
You have to continue living.

Once she settled in, Caridad focused on staying healthy and looking for new opportunities. She applied for welfare and found an affordable daycare center for her son. Though her English was rudimentary, she began taking a computer class in hopes of finding a secretarial job. She also began collaborating with Nini to find better health care. Caridad flourished under Nini's mentorship and succeeded in creating important alliances with a psychologist, various social workers, and a physician.

Julia

As my study progressed, I had the opportunity to visit a social service agency near Juana's apartment where I met Julia, a fifty-one-year-old activist and caseworker there. Julia had been born in Puerto Rico and had moved to the mainland in her youth. She agreed to work with me but was very hesitant to discuss sensitive topics such as her acquisition of the virus.

I used to be real open. I'm still open but I just choose when . . . A lot of
times I don't even talk about it. 'Cause, I definitely feel there's more to
me than a person living with HIV and that's not, not all of me. And that's
not the important thing in me.

Ironically, Julia was quite famous for her local advocacy work and had received many awards. Her wide social network gave her a great deal of influence in the HIV/AIDS community. Julia did feel comfortable explaining that she began this career as a recovering addict at a Latino social service agency. While there, she met Anita, a woman who spearheaded an important HIV/AIDS community-based organization (CBO) in the city. Anita took Julia under her wing, helping her thrive and encouraging Julia to follow her dreams:

> I was in [a small social service agency], I didn't want to go nowhere. And Anita opened the door to my house, she took me to my house, and it was a wonderful experience I guess from there on . . . she was running [an important HIV/AIDS organization] . . . she took me to my appointments and my social security and all the process, you know. And when we arrived at my appointments and I gave them my name . . . and they were like "Sit over there" [waving dismissively], you know . . . but when I arrived with Anita, its like, all doors opened, and she introduced me to a lot of people so that that I . . . could be connected, you know, so it was good.

Anita's connections meant that Julia could now get the help she needed without waiting, like everyone else. In time, Anita even began helping Julia start her own health-related social service projects. Julia's broad cultural capital helped her find powerful allies like Anita and excel at HIV/AIDS outreach. It gave her entry into many of Newark's ethnic communities. It also helped her access important resources:

> The reverends from the . . . church [have] been coming here, they pray with me, like for Thanksgiving they always send me this box of things . . . they got a list of names, people they pray for and always my name is there. I think it has to do with me staying healthy. They always been so good to me. And there's a male reverend and a female reverend, and she was the one that got me that little computer that I had here. When Reverend K. comes and lays hands on me, and she prays with me . . . it makes me feel so good.
>
> I used to go to this lady in Manhattan with a friend who went every month to be treated with crystals . . . and I used to love that. The lady would treat me for free. My friend used to pay bad money, seventy-five dollars an hour or something like that. And she used to do it for free, for me.

Julia soon realized how often she was treated differently from most of her HIV-positive friends and social service clients. She also realized the great impact this had on her life. "I never really have to wait too long to get an appointment. Not really. Because they know me. But other people that I talk to, they do go through a lot. . . . Sometimes I feel like I am so lucky and I know so much people and, and things get done, you know, for me that wouldn't get done [for other people]." However, Julia's broad social network came with disadvantages as well. Her many roles in the community created a heavy set of responsibilities. She was a public speaker, a case manager, a Narcotics Anonymous (NA) sponsor, and a mentor to many HIV-positive women and men. Finally, Julia faced constant pressure to maintain her sobriety regardless of the demands placed on her.

And though her cultural- and social-capital toolkit was broad, she had none of the organizational skills that her middle-class colleagues took for granted. Her desk was always buried under piles of unpaid bills—not because she had no money, but because she found it difficult to categorize, track, and pay them. She had been given a PC, but had no experience using Microsoft Office or Microsoft Word.

> You know, like, I need to start planning, if I have a follow-up appointment and I have to do something, and to prioritize things like go[ing] to Legal Aid and stuff to a lawyer for legal . . . if I keep putting it off when June 11 is here [and] I haven't done that . . . in voicemail there are thirty messages saved.

Shortly after we met, Julia left her job as a case manager to work as a pharmaceutical consultant. Ostensibly, she would be a traveling AIDS educator, but her real job was to promote a drug used to treat an HIV-related condition. Julia had used this drug with great success, and the company that produced it had seen the marketing potential of hiring her to advertise this in her home community.

The shift from community advocate to pharmaceutical consultant opened the door to a good salary and a better economic future. After years of volunteering for countless organizations, Julia had no savings, no retirement fund, minimal job security, and a very modest salary. Yet she was surrounded by middle-class professionals with good salaries, houses, health insurance, and job security. This looked like an opportunity to join them. But the company had hired her on a trial basis only; if she could not generate enough business for them, they would not keep her. They were also withholding health insurance, which she desperately needed.

The job required her to call contacts and set up appointments to conduct workshops. Then she had to arrange for catering and teach the workshops themselves. This meant creating lists of actual and potential clients, keeping detailed records of phone conversations, saving and organizing travel receipts, tracking gas mileage, and filling out reimbursement forms. Nothing in her past had prepared her for this; she had never even heard of a day planner when we met. Unfortunately, no one at the pharmaceutical company had thought to train her in the basic skills required for a white-collar sales job. From the outside, she seemed more than capable. How could they understand that the cultural capital that had helped her out of the "underclass" was insufficient to anchor her to the middle class? They neither understood, nor did they prepare her adequately. But they did protect themselves from the possibility of her failure.

Deborah

Julia introduced me to Deborah, a determined thirty-eight-year-old woman who had been born and raised in Newark. Deborah had pulled herself out of home-lessness, physical abuse, and addiction through sheer willpower and the help of several social workers. She showed me scars made by men who beat her up during her time on the street (see Romero-Daza 2005 for more about violence encountered by sex workers). Deborah thought she might have contracted HIV through IV drug use, but she wasn't sure. When we met she was living in a small one-bedroom apartment with her nineteen-year-old daughter.

> I was homeless for four years, with the virus and no health care. I was homeless with a teenage daughter. Living out of cardboard boxes . . . I was active [in addiction] . . . I was turning tricks to have food for my daughter and I . . . I ate out of McDonald's garbage can and everything. Panhandled. Lived in Penn Station bathroom in Newark. When I became homeless my daughter went to live with her dad, but it didn't turn out OK so then she came to stay with me and I was homeless. So I had her one day in my mother's house, one day in my sister's house and her grades were going down. So that's when I said, "I'm gonna try my best to get an apartment" and that's what I did, you know? I didn't go into detox. I cleaned myself, myself. I was clean already for two years before I got the apartment, on my own, I was going to [NA] meetings and stuff. I tried to stay in my sister's house until I . . . gather everything together like my paperwork and stuff like that. It took me two years.

Over the following two years, Deborah generated tremendous opportunities out of very little. She was eager to get off welfare and get a job. She started by volunteering at the small local hospital where she received medical care. Because she felt comfortable with the *habitus* of the middle-class professionals around her, she was able to seek out new information, advocate for herself, and settle into the hospital routine, making herself indispensable. "Like a lot of times they'll call me so I can go interpret because they don't have someone in the emergency room or they don't have someone on another floor."

After eight months, Deborah applied for a part-time job at the hospital and got it. She remained very actively engaged there, even confronting staff about HIV-related discrimination. At the same time, she was able to leverage her facility with the hospital environment by creating good relationships with doctors, nurses, and nonclinical staff. She even forged strong relationships with hospital administrators and directors. Every time she applied for a job, her friends and allies wrote her letters of recommendation. Eventually, Deborah began seeing her physician friends for regular and HIV-related care.

> It's good to always have a network of people that you know that can help you. And if they have a problem that they're going through, I always try to help [them] find a solution, too. I don't know. For some reason, I'm good with that. One of the doctors came up to me and he told me, "I want to refer you for in the emergency room, for receptionist, they need somebody." The doctor gave me a referral and you know, like a reference letter and stuff. . . . Let me tell you, [another] doctor gave me a hug and a kiss, and he told me, "You have a beautiful Christmas. God is going to bring you everything you need, Deborah." I mean, I was stunned, for him to give me a kiss first of all, on my cheek, and a hug . . . and my co-workers were like, yeah, everybody loves you around here . . . and the ladies that work on the cafeteria, they all know me already, they are like, "What's up Deborah? How are you doing? How are you feeling, Deborah?"

In other words, Deborah used her broad toolkit of cultural and social capital to create a powerful network that gave her emotional support, better economic opportunities, and more personalized medical care. In a little over a year and a half, she moved from homelessness to welfare, and from welfare to a full-time job and continuity of care.

Celestina

In New Brunswick, a clinic social worker introduced me to Celestina, a warm thirty-seven-year-old woman born and raised in Puerto Rico. Celestina spoke English but usually preferred Spanish. Both she and her husband Roberto were HIV-positive; he had unknowingly passed the virus to her during the course of their marriage. The discovery had crushed him as much as it had shocked her, and he struggled with ongoing feelings of sadness and guilt. But Celestina accepted this terrible turn of events with remarkable equanimity, deciding to do the best she could for her family. Together, the couple decided to leave Puerto Rico to get access to cutting-edge HIV treatments. They were strongly motivated to stay healthy so they could raise their two young sons. They also believed that the boys could benefit from greater opportunities on the mainland. So they packed up their children, along with very few belongings, and moved into the East Brunswick apartment above Roberto's sister and her husband.

Celestina was a kind soul, eager to "adopt" any stray person in need of a help. Her home became an after-school refuge for her son's schoolmates, and she fussed over them like a den mother. Celestina also offered her support to others attending her ID clinic, keeping an eye on young people with advanced HIV disease. The clinic staff soon noticed and began unofficially recruiting her help.

> While we are waiting at the clinic, Marco [a nurse] lowers his voice and asks in Spanish if Celestina can do him a favor. He tells her about a Mexican woman who speaks no English who has just been diagnosed positive. Carefully, he says that he would like her to think about this, but there is no pressure and she doesn't have to tell him now—would she consider allowing Marco to give the woman Celestina's phone number? Celestina is already interrupting him before he can finish, reassuring him that of course he can give out her number. Marco repeats that there is no reason for her to feel obligated. Celestina glances at Roberto and asks if it is OK—he says of course—and in Spanish she says "Yes, please tell her to call us." Marco says she doesn't know anything . . . could Celestina start explaining things to her and educating her? "Of course," she says, "of course." "This woman's family thinks that she is going to die tomorrow," says Marco. "You know how it is at first, you think that you are going to die right away."

CELESTINA: "No, but why? Haven't you told them?"

MARCO: "You know how it is . . . I tell her but it goes in one ear and out the other. She doesn't listen to me, but to you . . ."

CELESTINA: "It's different with us, you don't have it and she could think that you are just saying this to reassure her . . . I will talk to her . . ." (Field note 1999)

Celestina worked hard to maintain a positive attitude despite her illness, Roberto's advanced disease, and her many family responsibilities. Although she was well connected with diverse friends, staff, and social workers, she functioned as Roberto's primary source of support. She cheered him up when he felt depressed—a common occurrence—and urged him to keep fighting when he got sick—which was quite often. It was she who made his appointments and called the clinic when he was ill. Celestina also managed her sons' medical care and applied for the family's social security and welfare benefits. Through the clinic, she found the social service agencies that could provide the resources her family needed, and she was also the one who ferried her children to all of their extracurricular activities. When I asked her how she managed to do all of this, she told me:

> I enjoy it. I was about to start studying to become a nurse when I had to move here because of HIV. I would have liked it. I always ask a lot of questions. I want them to explain everything to me. When I see Dr. Patel, I ask her to explain exactly what [my problems] are and how I can prevent them. She explains them to me.

Once I visited the couple in the ER while both were being examined for potential opportunistic infections. On my way to their room, a nurse stopped me and told me that I needed to put on a gown and mask. When I asked him why, he hesitated and explained that they had not yet received a diagnosis—it was best to be careful. I was impressed that he maintained confidentiality regarding the couple's HIV status, but when I arrived gowned and masked, Celestina frowned at me in annoyance:

> The ER staff here is ignorant. They shouldn't make you wear all that stuff. We know more than they do. When Roberto got Cryptococcus and I heard that it could cause meningitis, I got scared for my children. So I asked Dr. Patel. She explained that the meningitis from Cryptococcus is different. It can't be spread by contact. And the doctors that come in here [her isolation room] don't wear that stuff [in fact, they did not]. They know. But these people, we know more than they do!

Celestina continued to live in East Brunswick for a year and a half after I met her, eventually succumbing to her overwhelming burdens and falling into her own depression. She struggled with recurrent illness and feared the side effects of HIV medications. Her family's food stamp allotment was repeatedly slashed and their tiny monthly check shrank until survival was impossible. Unlike others around her, Celestina refused to hide one smidgen of income or lie about her circumstances in any way. Even though their welfare benefits were pitiful and she and her husband had contributed to the system through paycheck withholding for decades, she did not feel entitled to one penny more than the law allowed. This was a serious problem, since welfare dispensed according to the letter of the law can rarely sustain a family's survival without supplementation (Sharff 1998). When her sister-in-law's family decided to move back to Puerto Rico, Celestina and Roberto decided to join them. They had learned that newer HIV drugs were being used on the island, and they already knew that the cost of living would be much lower there. Finally, both missed their families and the support they could provide.

Nerina

Most of the women who worked with me lived in Newark, but a few lived in the neighboring city of Elizabeth or a little further away, in New Brunswick. Nerina had been born and raised in New York City, but now lived in Elizabeth. I met her at an HIV/AIDS conference in Newark. Her bright pink jumper was accentuated by so many bracelets that I thought she might collapse beneath them. Her slender frame was covered in jewelry and she carried a cane, a huge purse, a fanny pack, a cell phone, and a beeper. At fifty-one, Nerina moved faster with her cane than I did without one. Fully loaded, she scampered along lightly while I struggled to keep up with her.

Nerina was an avid user of complementary and alternative medicine (CAM). As a strict vegetarian, she carried food with her at all times and rarely ate out, supplementing organic munchies with vegetarian cafeteria fare. Nerina carried agua de coco (coconut water), rice cakes, all-natural cookies, and tea bags of various kinds. She also loved the occasional Häagen Dazs bar. "I don't like protease inhibitors [HIV treatment drugs]. I worry about the side effects, 'cause they're all chemicals, and I'm not a chemical person. I'm more of a spiritual person. I'm more into Mother Nature. I'm not into science and all that stuff."

Nerina had not always been so health conscious; she believed she had acquired the virus while using drugs, doing sex work, and living on the streets of New York, although her understanding of the event that infected her was somewhat unorthodox. One day, she agreed to trade the use of her pipe for a hit of cocaine. While her friend was loading the delicate cylinder, he cracked it, cutting his finger. A tiny drop of blood dripped into the screen, but they smoked the pipe anyway.

> When he put my hit in there and I hit it . . . and I inhaled it . . . I felt the blood crystallize with the coke and it hit my lungs. I said, "What did I do?" I knew right then. Couple weeks later, they told me, "What's the matter with you? You look different! You look like you got the package ["package" was local slang for HIV at the time]." And I said, "But what are you talking about?" Because I was thinking to myself I'm not doing any more drugs than I normally do. You know what I'm saying? I'm not eating any less. So then the people kept telling me, like around a month, I got scared. I left a note on the van that used to come around and see the girls [the HIV/AIDS mobile testing van], and says I need to see you. There's something wrong. 'Cause I used to test every four months. And all of a sudden they called me up and they said, "Listen, we have to see you. Come downstairs and we'll talk to you." They don't say nothing over the phone.

This was one of many traumatic experiences in Nerina's life. As a child, her mother had abandoned her to an orphanage. Throughout her youth, she moved in and out of institutional settings and experienced sexual, emotional, and physical abuse at the hands of her father and others. Nerina never finished high school, but she did learn a great deal about institutions, bureaucracies, and the professionals who run them. Nerina was very good at telling middle-class professionals what they wanted to hear. Her extensive social network and broad cultural capital made it easy for her to work the system, but she usually did so to help others who needed it more than she. Of course, this skill also came in handy when she needed help: "Yeah, I go to legal aid, she does all that for me. I always go to her, and she does the paperwork, she's real good, at legal aid services. Ryan White pays for it. [The Ryan White Care Act is the largest single source of HIV care and service funding in the U.S.] I get it for free. And she was a director, and she said, 'I'm gonna write them my name and everything and if anything is a problem have them call me.'"

> When I broke my foot, I went up and saw Dr. Hamilton. I said, "I'm in a splint. What am I gonna do?" So he called up the number they gave me and it was closed. They had just closed. . . . But then there was this one doctor he knew, and she said, "I'll take of her." I first had to go downstairs, get registered, get the X-rays, and then go back to her. She said, "Do you know your foot is fractured in two places? Well, we gonna have to put a cast on you." And right away they put a cast on me.

Nerina volunteered at a small HIV/AIDS resource center, and helped new agency clients acclimate to a life with HIV. She also helped organize an HIV support group. Every day she left her house on foot and went to work at the agency, or made the rounds of her clinic appointments. She did not like to stay home, both because it bored her and because her husband had a serious alcohol problem that sometimes erupted into violence. "My old man, he's a pain in the ass [chuckling]. He never has time to do anything for me . . . [last week] he broke the mirrors. He was in jail and then, they had a paper that he couldn't come around, so he was staying at his friend's house. I don't know, he went crazy." Nerina preferred to be out in the community whenever possible, where she could spend time with her many friends and enjoy their emotional support. In return, she offered support to anyone who seemed to need it.

Selma

Nerina introduced me to Selma, a shy, thirty-one-year-old woman who also volunteered with her. She had been born and raised in Elizabeth, and took her recovery from (non-IV drug) addiction very seriously. Initially, Selma was reluctant to talk to me. She kept to herself, regarding me with suspicion. But after a few weeks, she began to relax and tell me a little about her life. Like many of the other women I worked with, Selma had experienced trauma and sexual violence. She was very careful about whom she trusted. "I don't trust anybody no more. I can't, I don't want, I can't seem to fall in love. You know the right way. 'Cause I got the virus and cause I know that's . . . why I got the virus. The virus was from falling in love."

And as a single mother of five, she had many responsibilities in addition to protecting herself and managing her health. Selma's ex-husband lived in Puerto Rico and offered her little assistance. Her current partner was living in a halfway house far away and could offer only emotional support. But it was he who had connected her to the HIV resource center when she tested positive for the virus.

> When I got the virus, [John] was already . . . with the virus and he was already coming here, to the resource center. And the resource center

recommended me, they told me to go for help. . . . I went to the doctor, and everything just fell into place. Everybody where I go knows about the virus. Everybody where I go, you know, have been compassionate toward the virus.

Over time, I watched Selma blossom: she learned everything she could while volunteering, making herself indispensable. She had completed her high school equivalency exam and taken short vocational school courses, acquiring useful work experience along the way. Consequently, the work habits and general *habitus* of middle-class organizations were comfortable for her. Selma enjoyed working, and quickly settled into the resource center routine. She also applied the strategies used to manage paperwork there to her own health care management. "I keep a record of everything. It has my blood work, my blood tests and I keep it here. I have copies of everything. Even copies of my bills."

Selma was comfortable with her ID-clinic doctor, although she did not get along with her family physician. Despite the fact that her clinic doctor did not have a strong reputation in the HIV community, she established a good rapport with him, and her health remained good. So Selma used most of her broad cultural capital to forge alliances across various agencies, drawing on resources offered by all of them. She was especially drawn to support groups. Eventually, she helped to establish a long-running, widely attended support group of her own. "In the last year I went to a women's support group held at the [agency], I do the Tuesday and Thursday morning support groups. Now we're trying to organize a new group on Monday nights, for everybody, not just women. Support groups are great." Over time, Selma's support group flourished. Since she was satisfied with her care and the emotional support of her network, she focused most of her attention on finding a job. Eventually, she succeeded in this as well, transitioning into a paid position at another social service agency.

Gabrielle

Gabrielle was another patient at the New Brunswick clinic. She thought she had contracted HIV from IV drug use, although she had also been exposed through sex work. In many ways this tall, wiry woman was both loving and tender. But her journey to a place of nurturance had been hard. She had experienced physical, sexual, and emotional abuse as a child in Puerto Rico. Twenty of her fifty-one years had been spent in prison. She had lived on the streets of both New York and Newark.

For me, you know, six years is not a lot . . . but when you spend time in jail, times are not long. You know, twenty years is long, thirty years, I mean there is a woman who does fifty. I did twenty years but when I came out I went back in again. . . . People [in jail] don't talk about having sex on the street for money. You don't say those things, you know. They was always a big dealer . . . but by me saying that, that I did, it opened the minds of other people.

Gabrielle worried that she had lived her life selfishly, inflicting harm on others. She worried about how her actions had impacted her children. She believed that her inconsistent parenting had shaped her son's indifference toward his own daughter, causing him to abandon the girl to her mother's whims after his divorce. Having been sexually molested as a child, Gabrielle was afraid when her granddaughter was left in the care of strangers. She constantly struggled with feelings of guilt, anxiety, and sorrow. Yet she actively protected her son's young daughter, and when she told her story, it revealed many examples of advocacy, generosity, and courage:

> I think I was the first person [in jail] that say in public I'm HIV . . . other people started coming out and now HIV is alright in jail. You know, but before people were very scared. And I was at the time, I used to be help-ing a nun. She and I used to wait for the buses to come with the new girls, right, and I tell them, "Look my name is Gabrielle and I'm an HIV person, if you need a person to talk to, just look at me, and I'll find you," and I did. The police would let me go to any floor, any room because they knew that I was going there talking to people, you know. I think that helped people! Make me more strong, and make me a better person. Eh . . . we made the first support group, it was like in an office. I was the first one in there . . . in the beginning, sick people was treated very bad in jail . . . very bad. Matter of fact, after I came out of jail a lady reverend went to the jail to make a speech and invited me too. That was nice. They invited me to talk to my friends. And as a matter of fact I'm thinking of going back so they could know that ten years later I'm still alive, and that they got hope.

Although Gabrielle had never completed high school, she had decades of experience in manipulating institutions. She had also encountered women of every background and social class in prison. "I met all kinds of people . . . everyone . . . even that lady that killed the doctor that made that book, the diet book . . . and I used to clean the church. I had a very good time. I worked as a drug counselor, too." Consequently, Gabrielle knew how to build connections with people of different backgrounds. She knew how to find the resources to survive and never hesitated to put this experience to good use. "I got everything before I came out of jail. 'Cause I was the type to work the program. I was responsible for me first. I had everything, everything! Room, everything! My SSI, everything. When I came out of jail the next day I had a hotel and every-thing. I get what I want." And in fact, she usually did.

Gabrielle was able to cross out of her *habitus* and forge boundary-spanning relationships, but she struggled to hold on to them. At the clinic, for example, she had both committed allies and vocal enemies among the staff. Her broad cultural capital was useful, but there were gaps in her ability to meet others' expectations. "You see I cry a lot, and people don't like it. I don't care. Because I'm taking all my anger, all my sadness away. If I keep them inside I get sick, Mami. I go crazy." Perhaps because of this struggle, she was very appreciative of the support her friends and allies offered:

> Support is very important, mama. Without support, you can't go on. You see, I know a lot of people that are sick, what they don't tell. They don't tell their kids, they don't tell nobody. And, that . . . stop them from having, taking care of themselves good. There's a lot of people that doesn't go to the hospital . . . they don't want people to know. That's weird!"
>
> When I go in Dr. Jeff, I like the man, he's very smart, a little crazy but he's very smart. And I take his advice, but always . . . we gonna do a little bit his way, and a little bit of mine. And he always says, "Let's do one of Gabrielle's things." Because he knows that I know what is good for me. You know what I'm saying, mama? Most of the time the doctors tell me what to eat but then from what the doctor tells me I gets my own opinion, a little bit of them and a little bit of mine makes it perfect. And I run always my life. I tell them what I do, what I need to be done, and most of the time they treat you very well.

Some of Gabrielle's most important allies helped her manage her health. She maintained very good relationships with her doctor and several clinic nurses, establishing a collaborative, team-based approach to her own care. Because of this, Gabrielle was able to manage her health in a way that brought her a measure of peace and satisfaction.

Average Cultural and Social Capital: Carlotta, Flor, Nilsa, Paquita, Amelia, Cristina, and Juana

Carlotta

When I met her, Carlotta was thirty-nine years old. She had been born and raised in Puerto Rico and had contracted HIV from her husband, who had a history of drug use. She had come to the United States in her early thirties hoping to further her high school education. She had taken some college-level classes, though she had never completed a college degree. Carlotta often struggled to fit her communication style with those of institutional and bureaucratic gatekeepers.

> As for me, I always, since I came to this country, I always tried to study and still when I was living in Puerto Rico, I wanted to study. What happens is that there I did not have people who, who helped me. I came here

because of that. And here I studied, that's why I say that there are people who think that I am somewhat dumb, or stupid, or lazy, but I don't have to, I don't have to ask a lot to understand things.

Carlotta was also uncomfortable operating in English, especially when she was nervous. When possible, she preferred to speak Spanish. Most of her books were in Spanish, and so were her favorite TV and radio programs. Although she had lived in Newark's multicultural environment for some years, her small network of friends was composed almost entirely of Puerto Ricans and a few Latin American immigrants.

When Carlotta and I met, Nini was helping her make appointments at various social service agencies in an attempt to help her secure better housing, free food vouchers, and energy-bill assistance. Nini also counseled Carlotta about the benefits of switching doctors and tried to show her how to acquire allies and get better care at their clinic. The mentoring process was not easy. Nini's strategy involved assessing the background and preferences of each potential ally and tailoring her approach to that person accordingly. This was especially difficult for Carlotta, who could not mimic Nini's flexible approach.

For example, although Carlotta shared Nini's strong distaste for drug use and promiscuity, she did not discuss her husband's role in her misfortune or emphasize her disapproval of drugs. She did not try to signal respectability by dressing conservatively. If she was excited, she raised her voice; if she was angry, she showed it freely. In other words, Carlotta did not attempt to tailor her behavior to the expectations of clinic and agency personnel. Like most people, she could not cross out of her native *habitus* with ease. While this should have had no impact on the quality of care that she received, it did. Because physicians and clinic staff were sometimes uncomfortable around her, they interacted with her less frequently, investing less in her well-being. Sometimes these encounters even became hostile.

> Yes, she treated me a little poorly and I answered her because supposedly, as I say, supposedly at the clinic the boss is the doctor, isn't he? Then if I am sick and the doctor says, "Tell Miss Lopez to come talk to me on such day." Then the doctor has more authority than the receptionist, then that is what she did, acting stupid there and I said "No, but the doctor sent for me." And she . . . "Ay, I don't care. You're not supposed to be here." Then we ended up arguing and she called the security guard on me.

Nevertheless, Carlotta's ongoing struggle with institutional settings did not discourage her from trying to take care of herself. She simply shifted to brief, early morning appointments that minimized her time at the clinic and put most of her energy into complementary and alternative modalities that she could control herself. Carlotta drank herbal teas, took vitamins, and performed spiritual self-healings, pursuing any easily available CAM modality that seemed useful. She also began listening to a Spanish radio program that emphasized spiritual approaches to health maintenance. In this way, she limited the time she spent outside her own *habitus* while managing her symptoms and the side effects of the drugs she was prescribed.

Flor

Through Nini, I also met Flor, Nini's thirty-nine-year-old ex-sister-in-law. Flor had been born in Puerto Rico and had come to Newark as a young woman. Her first husband, Nini's brother, had spent many years as an IV drug user early in the epidemic. He contracted HIV and died many years before Nini acquired the virus. Flor did not believe that she had acquired the virus from him, however. She thought she had acquired it from her second partner, although she might also have been exposed through a prior addiction. Regardless, Flor was more fortunate than either of her husbands: although she was HIV-positive, she had lived in good health for many years. Flor had never been symptomatic and had only decided to be tested after she discovered that her second partner was HIV-positive.

After Flor was diagnosed, she did not know where to go or what to do. She found herself reading flyers and folders related to HIV care wherever she found them posted, explaining that, "I kept on reading like papers and papers all over . . . I didn't know what I was looking for, a clinic or a hospital . . . I didn't know, I never . . . because I didn't know where to go or ask." Consequently, it was some time before she was connected to a regular source of HIV care.

When Flor finally found a clinic, she was referred to several social service agencies that could provide her family with significant support. Although she was most comfortable with her own small network of Puerto Rican friends and relatives, she did forge a few outside partnerships, mostly with social workers. One of Flor's daughters had been born with birth defects and required a great deal of care. The social worker at her clinic arranged for regular professional home care. At first, the agency sent different workers on different days. This proved uncomfortable for Flor, who wanted to establish an ongoing relationship with a single individual.

> In the beginning they was changing, but I told them, I said, you know, don't keep changing, just one nurse for my daughter, because when a new one came I had to show them where food at, where the bathtub and everything, show them how to feed her. But Brenda, she knows, you can count on her, do anything, she know what time her appointments, you know.

Flor's family was large: she, her seven children, and her current husband lived together in a large, run-down apartment in a shabby part of the city. She was pregnant when we met and was eventually put on AZT. In clinics and hospitals, Flor stayed quiet. She did not feel comfortable with most of the professionals around her, and this made it difficult for her to advocate for herself. She struggled with a team of doctors who did not communicate well among themselves: her OB/GYN put her on one medication, but her ID clinic doctor switched it without warning. Caught between the two in an unfamiliar territory, she seemed uncertain about what to do: her native cultural capital had not prepared her for this challenge.

Nilsa

Nilsa, one of Nini's closer friends, lived in the public housing project at the far end of Nini's street. She had been born in Puerto Rico but had lived in Newark for over half of her thirty-nine years. Few of her friends and none of her neighbors knew that she was HIV-positive. Nilsa leaned heavily on Nini and her Pentecostal faith for support. She had contracted the virus from her husband, who had a history of multidrug use. He had tested positive in prison, while serving a six-year prison sentence. Initially, he told Nilsa about it, but later reversed himself, explaining that he had accidentally gotten someone else's test results. She believed him because she had been tested upon his incarceration and the results had been negative. Nilsa stayed celibate throughout their separation, thinking that she was safe from HIV. Shortly after his release they began living together again. On a hunch, she decided to get tested a few months later. When the test came back positive, she knew she had been lied to.

Nilsa frequently voiced the pain of being a "respectable woman" who had never courted HIV risk. She felt that she did not deserve what had happened to her. She had never used drugs and had always been monogamous. When I met her she was understandably angry, and her hostility sometimes spilled out on those around her. The traumas she had endured had created a fury she could barely contain. Her rage was matched only by frustration at the poverty that handicapped all her attempts to improve her family's life.

To make matters worse, Nilsa struggled to acclimate to the demands of the bureaucracies she depended on. She could not replicate Nini's repertoire of interactive styles. Health care professionals and social workers did not identify with Nilsa or feel impelled to help her.

She was constantly in conflict with the middle-class professionals she encountered, often with good reason. Sometimes she directed her frustration at those with the power to help her cut through roadblocks and red tape. She was often turned away by those who did not care to assist her and those with no patience for her anger.

> It hurt me a lot and all that, and then they sent me for, some ultrasound . . . when I went back over there a month ago they didn't have the results. And

I asked her, I said, "Yeah but you know what? I wanna have my tests results 'cause I want to know what I have in there, because to have a pain all the time, something is wrong, right?" Well, she took an attitude. She says, "Well, what do you want me to do? I can't do nothing! If you have anything to say, go out there at the front desk and tell *them*. But don't come with me!" You know, "Dudududu [mimics the doctor speaking with disrespect]."

And she's a doctor and she's treating me like that? And I say . . . I look at her and I get very upset and I ask her, "You know what? I am the one who's sick here. You're not sick. You're a healthy woman, thank God. And, if I don't worry about *mi salud* [my health], you ain't gonna do it, nobody else. I have to worry about it. You don't care because you don't know what's going on in here and you're not the one who's taking the pain. But I have to care because it's my life." . . . And she said, "Hmph! Well, like I said, if you have any complaints, go over there, tell them, but don't tell me. What do you want me to do? I already did what I could."

And I say, "Forget it, this is it! No more, no more! I'm not gonna take bullshit from nobody because I don't need it. You know? I don't need that aggravation from a doctor! You know, to treat me like that!" My Medicaid is paying her and she got a job because I am in this position right now. What's she gonna come and treat me like that then, no way! I'm not gonna go there no more . . . I go back, yes, for the last visit that is gonna be this month because I want to talk to . . . but if she comes and gets my record I'm not gonna let her see me. I'm gonna tell her right there in front of all the patients, "No, lady, I don't need the way you treat me. Put it back." You know? But I want to see if they give me a letter that I need, 'cause I'm trying to, to see if they can give me a better place that I can move, like I've been saying, you know?

During the time I spent with Nilsa, she continually complained about the injustices she had endured. She had good reasons to complain. Her HIV-related symptoms exacerbated her other problems. She saw a merry-go-round of physicians, rarely consulting the same doctor three times in a row. As was typical of the women in my study, Nilsa had to cope with too many things at once: poverty, poor health, and two teenagers—one developmentally disabled and the other an addict. She moved in and out of paralysis and exhaustion, unable to muster the strength to pursue more help.

But Nilsa's anger made case managers and health care professionals more likely to avoid her, making an already difficult path even thornier. And though she used her native cultural capital resourcefully—stretching her tiny budget and raising children in poverty—her expertise stopped there. Nini noticed Nilsa's lack of connection with resource gatekeepers and tried to help her. In the end, Nini did help Nilsa find better health care, but she could not transmit her broad cultural and social capital to her friend. Nilsa was never able to forge strong alliances with physicians or social workers while we worked together under Nini's tutelage.

Paquita

Nini introduced me to Paquita, a thirty-nine-year-old woman who had been born in Puerto Rico. Nini explained that Paquita was ill and very depressed. Paquita's many co-morbidities (obesity, stroke, HIV) made it difficult for her to leave her apartment. She managed her weekdays with the assistance of two home-health aids. She was married, but her husband worked all week. Nini visited Paquita periodically to see how she was doing but felt unable to help her; she worried that Paquita was fighting a losing battle to maintain her health and emotional stability.

When I met her, I understood why. At nearly three hundred pounds, Paquita found every kind of movement a challenge. Her weight and her difficulty controlling one leg kept her largely wheelchair bound. Paquita spent most of her time watching soap operas and I observed few visits from friends or family. Her daughter and granddaughter lived in another state and were rarely able to come see her. Paquita's poor health and isolation fueled a deep depression that dominated her life. She often broke into tears, wailing loudly in anguish. In truth, her life was very lonely.

> When I got this thing I was really scared. I'm losing my mind . . . sometimes I think I gotta go this way and then it's not. I gotta go the other way. I'm getting . . . pretty old. It gets me scared sometimes . . . being alone.
>
> I went to the emergency room [several months] before you came. . . . I went to the doctor for depression. My husband drove me. I wanted to stay in, but they sent me home. I was hoping they could help . . . worrying for death and for sickness, [but] they don't, they don't prefer me to go for that [depression].

Paquita had contracted HIV from a previous partner. It had moved quickly through her system, and in combination with obesity, had seriously compromised her health. Her husband, a conservative evangelical Christian, was HIV-negative. He helped take care of her but was not accepting of her illness, nor was he an advocate for her health. Their marriage was not a happy one, and their home was filled with tension and anxiety.

> I am angry, very angry . . . Last night Maria [the evening home-health aide] didn't come. The phone rang at seven o'clock but my husband wouldn't answer it. "It's too late, Paquita" [she mimics his voice]. He never wants to help me. It makes me so mad, so mad I want to do something to hurt him. . . . He *never* wants to do *anything* with me. He won't even kiss me. I tell him, "You won't get anything from kissing!" But he doesn't do it. It bothers me because I miss it. I miss it.

Paquita never became comfortable with the treatments and social services she received. Despite her long tenure at Nini's ID clinic and the home services she received, Paquita did not take an active interest in managing her health. She could never remember which agencies provided her with which resources, nor did she feel able to reach out and get more help—which may well have been related to the sadness and depression with which she struggled. And even though Paquita visited the ID clinic on a monthly basis, she seemed lost, not knowing exactly where to go or what to do whenever a new problem emerged.

> [About a large HIV agency:] They used to help me, but they didn't really support me. And now I don't know what's going on. I went for just a few months. I don't like it.
>
> I was going [to a mental health clinic] at the big hospital, once a week. But . . . the lady that was treating me, she started saying something I didn't like. So I left. I stopped.

This distant connection to health care professionals and social service personnel did not mean that Paquita never asked for help. For a time, she was visited by a kind, Caribbean physical therapist. Occasionally, a white, non-Hispanic counselor also came to see her. I saw her ask them for small items and help with minor tasks. But these relationships remained distant. Paquita frequently asked me to take dictation so she could write letters to friends and relatives in Puerto Rico. Talking about these relationships gave her the greatest joy and brought the most animation to her face.

On most of my visits, Paquita requested small items for my next trip: gifts for her granddaughter, inexpensive perfumes, or little treats. It felt good to be able to cheer her in small ways, and I suspect that her therapists sought similar comfort. But these exchanges never seemed to evolve into strong ongoing bonds. Even Paquita's home-health workers, whom she saw every weekday, seemed eager to leave the moment a potential replacement arrived.

I also noticed that most of the time, Paquita did not get good-quality care. The medical consultations I observed were brief and desultory. Her doctors seemed rushed. They did not show any particular interest in her case other than that which was absolutely required. This was particularly striking when I compared her care to the care I saw offered to others less in need. But Paquta was in no position to advocate for herself, and as far as I could tell, no one else did it either.

Amelia

Through Julia, I met Amelia, a gentle thirty-eight-year-old woman who had been born and raised in Newark. She, her husband, Pedro, and their two children all lived in a tiny efficiency apartment. Their only bathroom was shared with her husband's relatives, who lived in the apartment upstairs. Both Amelia and Pedro were HIV-positive, but the children, born from Amelia's previous marriage to an intravenous drug user, were HIV-negative. Amelia was tested for the virus after her divorce, when she decided to enter the hospital for a tubal ligation. She eventually discovered that her ex-husband had been admitted to the hospital years before with HIV-related ailments and put two and two together, though he never told her he had the virus.

> In the beginning, when I found out, I went to a support group. Yeah, now, I talk to nobody. Yeah, it was like we all get together, we share a story, we tell our, you know, good and bad things. . . . I went . . . like a year, and then the program finished. I think that's what really helped me a lot, you know what I'm saying? It made me realize that I'm not alone, you know, to see there's people like me. You know, and we share, we share a lot. And we keep in touch on the phone. They were pretty good. But today? I don't think so. I mean . . . I'm not a person that really . . . likes to express my feelings too much. And I like more to myself. I like to keep away, keep away, I guess. I'm always home with my kids, you know what I'm saying? I mean like right now I'm OK I don't feel like I need it, you know what I'm saying?

Amelia was tender, compassionate, and shy. She often felt sad, preferring to stay at home. She spent long periods of time sleeping and crying in isolation. Still, she was always willing to talk or emerge from her home if she thought someone needed her help. When it came to helping herself, though, the situation was different.

> Nobody can help me. You know, I mean I feel like nobody can help me. I mean, sometimes, I don't even know what's going on with me, you know what I'm saying? . . . At times I've been depressed, at times I've been confused. Most of the time I'm confused. I don't know which way to go, when coming and going, like about my bills, I know I put it someplace, and this is causing me problems, I don't where I put 'em at. For myself I would've give up. Yeah, I would've given up. But I know I have two kids there so I have to live for them because I know they need me, OK, 'cause I'm their mother. And their father, I think it's, you know, Pedro is not their real father. You know what I'm saying? So I'm both to them. And I am, you know, confused about it. I'm more to myself.

When Amelia did seek help outside of her family and close friends, she experienced persistent discomfort. Even when she liked individual social workers or health care professionals, she could not forge strong bonds with them. Thus, her social circle remained small, and only the most persistent outsiders could get in.

> I like to keep away, keep away, I guess. I'm always home with my kids and, you know what I'm saying? I used to go to [an agency] for marriage

counseling. I was having a lot of problems and was under a lot of pressure and I was under a lot of pressure, and then we went to talk to the . . . person, and it was good talking to her because she was real nice and everything. But I feel like, like I was wasting my time, you know what I'm saying? I mean she was real nice, real beautiful but, it just . . . I felt uncomfortable. And so, I didn't go back.

Amelia's preference for her small social circle meant that she seldom ventured out of her comfort zone. When she did go out, her husband usually accompanied her. She depended on him to keep the family abreast of social services offerings, and to mediate between her and those professionals whom she could not escape.

To tell you the truth I just go in, do what we gotta do, that's it and get out. I'm not a person that I'm gonna tell my doctor "I feel like this, I feel like this, I feel like this." No. Just take my blood and . . . I'm like that. I'm . . . I always been like that. And my husband go with me, I tell my husband, tell him I have this, tell him I have . . . my husband have to talk for me, 'cause I, I don't wanna talk!

I feel like they're doing their job and that's what they're there for, you know, I haven't found a person that I can feel comfortable with . . . you know what I'm saying? So like [the social worker at her clinic], I don't feel comfortable with him, I'm sorry! I know he's nice . . . but I can't, I just can't.

Above all, Amelia dreaded going to hospitals and clinics. She was especially uncomfortable with ID clinic physicians, whose questions sometimes implied promiscuity or drug use on her part. Because of this, she avoided her regular checkups for months at a time, even endangering her health. "You know, I hate to go to doctors, to the hospital, so I want to go to somewhere that's fast and quick and get it over with and take me home, you know? That's it. Give me what I need and that's it."

Amelia also hated the side effects of her HIV medications. They exhausted her and kept her from playing with her children. Amelia was repelled by the way the drugs made her arms and legs grow thinner while her belly swelled up. Understandably, these side effects kept her from fully embracing her treatment regimen.

Cristina

I met Cristina in New Brunswick through a clinic nurse. At thirty-two, she had spent many years grappling with drug addiction in Newark before moving to New Brunswick and Massachusetts. In 1989 she entered a drug-treatment program at a small Latino social service agency and tested positive for HIV. Eventually, she moved to Massachusetts and began working for an HIV agency there. But

Cristina wasn't able to maintain this life and was eventually incarcerated for four years. When I met her, she was attending a New Brunswick exit program that helped former prisoners in recovery find housing and get jobs. Despite her troubles, she was willing to share her insights about living with HIV.

Cristina was eager to "graduate" from her program, find her own apartment, and create a stable life so that DYFS (the Division of Youth and Family Services, responsible for child protection and welfare) would allow her to regain custody of her teenage son. She often talked about how much she missed him and searched tirelessly for an affordable apartment that that would provide him with his own room. But finding her place in the world was challenging without a social network. Her mother lived in Puerto Rico, her newer friends were all in Massachusetts, and her old friends were still struggling with active addiction. "I used to live in the projects here for awhile, when I was on the street. I went back and it was hard. All the people I did drugs with were there. If I want my son back, I have to stay away."

Although Cristina was determined to succeed, she was unsure of what to do with so little help and guidance. She searched unsuccessfully for an apartment for months, and whenever a new obstacle appeared, she felt paralyzed, powerless, and overwhelmed. Without local allies, Cristina seemed to spin her wheels, unable to gain traction in her quest. The professionals who might have helped her offered limited support, but she struggled to forge strong bonds with them. She believed that white middle-class people would not respect her, and her conflicted relationship with clinic staff and physicians reinforced that belief. Cristina was certain that her ethnicity and history of drug use stigmatized her in their eyes. Ultimately, she connected with only one kind but overworked Puerto Rican social worker:

> I feel so comfortable like when I'm talking to Rosita because I, she understands where I'm coming from . . . the way I am and whatever I just feel comfortable because, you know, I don't think I'm prejudiced, or anything, it's just that I feel comfortable with her. You know, and I talk to her in Spanish and I talk to her about music and, you know whatever, and I just don't feel as comfortable . . . sometimes I even feel inferior, and I hate to say that, but that's the way I feel sometimes. Like with the doctors and nurses, and, you know, and they're all American, you know, white Americans. And so I feel like they look down sometimes. I don't know if I'm wrong.

Cristina bonded most strongly with Latinos from similar backgrounds, with whom she felt a kinship. Maintaining alliances with the white and African American middle-class professionals proved too difficult, so she began avoiding clinics, agencies, and even the support group she had recently joined. Her exit program had offered temporary women's support groups and she had hoped to find similar relief from the clinic's HIV/AIDS support group. But shortly after joining, she quit. When I asked her why, she said,

> I just didn't feel comfortable. You know as far as like, to speak, I don't know if . . . some . . . if culture has to do with it? But there was no Spanish people there really [laughing]. So you know I just didn't feel comfortable. And then the doctor is the one that runs that support group. So if you have a, you know, a complaint you can't even say . . . you know you can't . . . it supposedly should be where you can speak about everything, and you just, you don't . . . feel like that, you don't feel comfortable, you know . . . like I said, your, culture and the way you live has a lot to do with how, you know, how you know a person. . . . Because everybody has different cultures, different ways of living. And, if you can understand where I'm coming from, you know, you can treat me better . . . you know, it's, like, it's hard to put into words.

Cristina eventually found an apartment and secured custody of her son. She met a man she liked who accepted her HIV status. Things seemed to be looking up until her brother was released from prison. When he moved in and began using drugs, Cristina started to worry about his influence on her son. The resulting stress manifested in relationship problems and conflicts with her child. And again, isolation added to her pain. When I asked her if she had anyone at all to talk to, she said, "No, no one. I just stay in the house all day." Before long, Cristina returned to drugs in response to her anxiety. Despite her deepest hopes, she found herself overwhelmed, with nowhere to turn.

Juana

I met Juana while helping a social worker deliver groceries in Carlotta's neighborhood. This curvaceous, thirty-seven-year-old woman lived with her young daughter. She had been born in Puerto Rico but had moved to Newark in her twenties. Juana discovered her HIV status when she entered the hospital for a tubal ligation, attributing her infection to a former boyfriend. The news marked the beginning of a very bad period.

> What happens is that at that time my mother died, in '93, and I discovered in '92 [that I was sick], all at the same time. Then with the death of my mother I became more depressed and everything. I became extremely nervous. I would get up in the early morning every day. I could not sleep. I would call the ambulance. And when I went to the hospital I asked myself what was the matter with me, because I didn't have anything! It was my nerves. The man I was living with had gone to his wife, whom he had brought from Santo Domingo. I discovered my problem in '92 . . . in February. . . . Then in March I began to go to the clinic, and in April came his wife. And in April he left and went to her. Everything happened at the same time!

He went to her because he had her in Santo Domingo while he had me here. Then he had the two of us. Then he had to bring her here. Then when he brought her, he went with her. Then now she found another man, then he is here with me. That's the way men are. And I did not want him here, but he insisted and insisted until he stayed. As he is the father of my daughter, you know. And the situation is not so good to be changing men and I don't know what.

This combination of events proved too much for her to bear, and she entered a long depression. Although she joined a support group, it was not enough to pull her out of an emotional tailspin. Juana began sleeping all day and isolating herself in her apartment, refusing to answer the phone or door. During this period she went out only to attend to her daughter, buy groceries, and go to work. Still, she developed useful strategies for managing her sadness. "When I am depressed, I better begin reading the psalms in the Bible. Or I begin to pray, asking Jehovah who gives health, strength to a person. That makes me feel better."

Prayer, biblical study, and spiritual healing proved excellent coping mechanisms; they gave her hope and eased her worries about raising her daughter alone. Juana's father and siblings lived in Puerto Rico, where she had been born. She could not lean on them in her daily life, but she did visit them for extended periods every summer. Juana looked forward to this with great excitement: "Ten months here with the same routine and because of that I go every year, every summer to Puerto Rico for two months. There I unload everything, all that depression . . . I feel fine when I see my family."

When we met, Juana was raising her daughter alone. She had become tired of the way her on-again, off-again partner Carlos lived off her small income, contributing nothing to the household. Although he had a job, he spent his money as he liked, staying out late and returning home with empty pockets. "And I am the one who supports me. All by myself!"

Juana was extremely frustrated with this state of affairs, but she worried about the effect of another separation on her daughter. Still, as a legally married man, Carlos could not marry her. This meant that she could not find full acceptance in the church she loved. Finally, she threw him out. A year and a half later, he returned. Juana found him a new job and insisted that he contribute toward household expenses. And though his return was part of a repeating pattern, she had high hopes of success. I could only hope she was right.

Somewhere in the Middle: Luchita and Alicia

Luchita

Luchita, a thirty-four-year-old home health worker, agreed to meet me on her lunch break. She had been born in Puerto Rico and raised in Newark since infancy. Luchita discovered her HIV-positive status when she entered the hospital to give birth to a daughter. There she learned that her husband had given her the virus. She divorced him and married a kind and caring HIV-negative man a few years later. Their family prospered as both parents worked very hard to support their six children.

Luchita had no health insurance and ADAP (the AIDS Drug Assistance Program, designed to ensure that uninsured HIV-positive individuals could access anti-viral medications) paid for her HIV drugs. Although she had applied for Medicaid, she had been denied coverage because her husband had access to health insurance through his work. However, he was only able to insure himself, so they enrolled the children in New Jersey's Kidcare program, the state's subsidized plan for uninsured children. The couple paid out-of-pocket for everything else. For many years, Luchita was unfamiliar with the resources available to the HIV community. It took her a long time to find specialized HIV care and connect with programs like ADAP.

In her case, this was less of a hardship than usual. Although she did not venture far from her home community, she had a very close relationship with a well-educated, knowledgeable, and supportive pastor who knew a great deal about HIV/AIDS. Her pastor pulled her into the church network, encouraged her to volunteer as a youth minister, and even collaborated with Luchita to bring AIDS education into the church's ministry.

> She speaks Spanish; she is Dominican. She was in the Catholic Church, but the priest threw her out because she was telling the truth. . . . She always says we have to help each other. I started going to church and she was helping me. She said the best thing was for me to get closer, so the church could help take care of the kids and me. Now my husband goes and my children go too. Then my pastor started seeing the way the youth call me. I don't go [to work with them] every Thursday but I go when I can. [And] I go to their houses and pray with them.

This supportive religious community, spearheaded by her activist pastor, was the bedrock of her family's life. It sustained them in times of trouble. Luchita did not seem to feel any of the depression, anger, or suspicion I so often encountered in women who had acquired HIV from secretive partners. Instead, she seemed joyful, talking often of her faith in God and the delight she took in her religious community's love.

> It is very different when you have God and then you have your brothers in church. They are very strong with you and the love, that's the most thing we always look for, [people] infected with AIDS, the most things we look for is for love, you know, cheerful moments and, you know, understanding and, all my brothers in Christ they know that I'm infected and they don't reject me. . . . They get mad at me 'cause sometimes they drink

from the cup and I be like, no, no . . . I can be drinking coffee and they just snatch it out of my hands. And I be like, no, no . . . they be like [feigns drinking it]. . . . When I'm at my pastor's house, she invite me over to eat . . . and all of a sudden she just come from nowhere, take my fork, pluck my meat out and [eating motion]. . . . One thing I could say for my pastor, she's very open to people with AIDS. She is very, very open.

Pastor Flores was also instrumental in making sure that Luchita received high-quality care. Although Luchita's social network was based entirely on one small Latino church, her well-connected, activist pastor stepped in as her advocate and ally whenever she needed help. This helped offset Luchita's weak connections with social workers, physicians, and allies outside of her church.

Like when I get admitted at the hospital, you know how your body feels so weak you can hardly talk? You know you cannot talk or, or sign papers or do anything. So what, what happened is my pastor and my sister from Jersey be there, and they ask the doctor why you giving her that medicine? What's the name of the medicines? What is the side effects of the medicine? Have they ever give her that before? *Why* are you giving her that? Why? And what are the side effects of that medicine? You know because when you in the hospital and you cannot talk you know they give you anything! They be like, "Oh let's try this one on her to see the result." Then the next morning they come and take blood work on you. I'm not stupid, you know. So that's why my pastor be *on them*. "Why are you giving her that? Don't give her nothing without my authorization!" Which I gave my pastor permissions. Why? Because I don't know what these people is giving me! I don't know if it is a new medicine and he is trying it out on me and then they come running in and want to take blood work from you, and see whether the medicine is working or not!

Luchita had another great advantage: her husband accepted her HIV status completely and worked hard in their home. He did over half the cooking and cleaning and he took on half of the couple's childcare responsibilities. His approach greatly enhanced Luchita's quality of life—compared to the other women I worked with, she was much less burdened. In return, she had nothing but praise for him. She often spoke about his hard work, support, and commitment to their children. Despite the challenges she faced, Luchita's successful marriage and her powerful church-based network sustained her with great success. Every time I saw her, she seemed to radiate joy.

When I asked about her positive attitude, Luchita told me that someone in her position couldn't be depressed all the time; it was important to avoid worrying in order to stay healthy and whole. She would often shake her head in perplexity when confronted with the depressions of her HIV-positive peers.

Alicia

Alicia, a slender thirty-four-year-old with three children, remained quiet in any group that did not include her few close friends and family. I met her at the preliminary meeting of a women's HIV support group, where she sat in absolute silence the entire time. But when the two of us walked back to her home, she overwhelmed me with her outspoken self-assurance and strong opinions. First she announced that she wouldn't waste her time going back ever again because too many people had complained about their lives. Then she told me that she had no interest in being around negative people, and too many people with HIV spent all their time complaining. When I stammered out my surprise at this outburst of frank opinions, she laughed at me. Then she explained that people outside of her family and friends always thought she was shy and reserved.

Later, when I asked why she avoided support groups and rarely attended community gatherings, she answered, "It's hard for me to say. It's that I don't know, ok, I understand it's a support group, you know, but I don't know, you know. It's like for me . . . it's like taking my business out, and I'm not that kind of person."

Alicia discovered that she was HIV-positive when she began experiencing puzzling physical conditions—her face and eyes swelled up to huge proportions for no reason, and an emergency room visit revealed that the culprit was toxoplasmosis. This diagnosis, common for those living with HIV but rare for anyone else, prompted an ER doctor to offer her an HIV test. The results came back positive. This was not a complete surprise. Although she had no history of drug use, her husband had been a longtime IV drug user. He had died a few years before, and Alicia knew he had put her at risk of acquiring the virus.

Yet she had not been tested, partly because she hated emergency rooms and hospitals, and preferred to stay close to home. Alicia even avoided social service agencies most of the time. But her husband's diagnosis had connected her to one small agency and, through it, a man who had lived with HIV for many years. Nelson was a well-known AIDS activist in the local African American community. He maintained a rich network of local connections in the HIV/AIDS community, and he went with Alicia to get her test results.

> I was with Nelson, and Nelson acted real quick. He knew about everything that was going on, so I knew about the clinic because of him . . . [then] Nelson told me to change my doctor . . . like the third, fourth or fifth day. . . . I was with Dr. Raymond which I haven't gotten along with him. So Nelson told me to try Dr. Bach and since then I've been with Dr. Bach. [Dr. Raymond] is not a doctor that you could sit down and talk to him and to explain to him and like. You know if you had something to say, "OK, how you doing, OK?" "I feel like this and this,". . ."OK, here is your prescription, OK, bye." Not Dr. Bach. Dr. Bach sits down and if he has to give you a new medication he'll explain to you the side effect, what

would happen, what could go wrong, everything, everything. He takes a while. He'll actually take two hours in a room and even if he explained to you and you don't understand, 'cause sometimes they explain to you and you don't understand, he goes all over again and you know he makes me feel comfortable with him.

TABLE 2.3

Overview of Women

	Average capital	In the middle	Broad capital
Total	7	2	8
Education			
Didn't finish high school	6	2	3
Some college/technical school	1	0	5
Other issues			
Partner living at home	4	1	4
Children at home	6	2	4
English fluency issues	2	0	2
Reported chronic HIV symptoms	3	0	2
Reported chronic medication side effects	4	1	0
Acute hospitalizations	2	1	3
Risk factors for HIV			
History of substance abuse	2	0	5
Reported sexual abuse	1	0	5
History of sex work	1	0	3
Reported domestic violence or threat of violence	2	0	5
Ability to form alliances			
Strong clinician alliances	1	1	6
Strong service alliances	1	1	6
Strong support group alliances	1	2	6
Outcome			
Success accessing economic resources	2	1	8
Success obtaining high-quality care	0	1	6

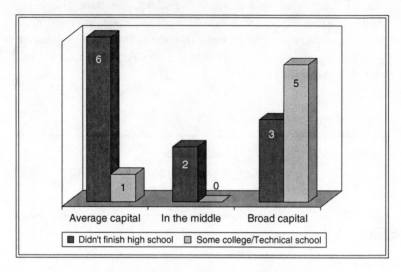

FIGURE 2.1 Education Level

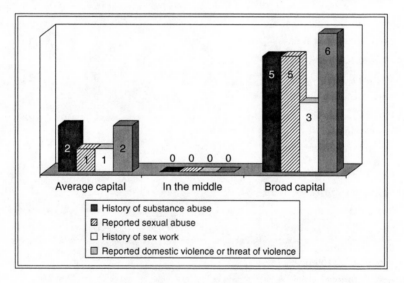

FIGURE 2.2 Risk Factors for HIV

Nelson also connected Alicia with social service and CAM treatment programs. Through her well-connected friend, Alicia found expert support in the HIV community and made friends who understood the challenges of raising children alone while managing HIV. However, her desire to stay close to home did not change. She built her network while spending most days at home watching over her daughters by following Nelson's advice and encouraging visitors.

Alicia's wish to stay home was strengthened by the side effects of her HIV medications. She resented them and often commented that she had felt fine until she started taking the drugs. Alicia was often exhausted, and emphasized that she now had to conserve her energy to meet the essential demands of parenting and daily life. "[I'm] constantly tired, my body aches. You know, I don't have like the energies to get up and go." On bad days, when she felt weak and ill, she would snuggle up in a comforter on the couch and rest until it was time for her children to come home from school. After Selma and her family moved in next door, Alicia spent more time socializing, but did not make any attempt to get out of the house more often.

Emerging Patterns

All the women in this study were subject to the kinds of structural violence that characterize the SAVA epidemic. Whether or not they had direct experience with drug use and sex work, all of these women were harmed by the SAVA complex of substance abuse, violence, and AIDS. Their lives were subjected to dangerous structural forces over which they had little or no control; all were preferentially exposed to the HIV virus (Connors 1996; Farmer, Simmons, and Connors 1996; Singer 1996). Many were also endangered by physical, emotional, and/or sexual abuse (Caridad, Deborah, Nerina, Gabrielle), placing them at additional risk for the virus (Romero-Daza, Weeks, and Singer 2003; Berger 2004; Romero-Daza, Weeks, and Singer 2005). Each woman struggled to protect herself and her family in this unforgiving environment.

All the women in this study made some attempt to reach out for help, whether or not they were able to find it in a form they could ultimately use. Women with average capital reached out for help, as did their counterparts with broad cultural and social capital. Most were able to establish at least one useful cross-*habitus* alliance that offered them important survival benefits, as in the case of Alicia (with Nelson), Luchita (with her pastor), Flor (with her daughter's caregiver), and Juana (with her infectious disease clinic doctor). A few depended on only one or two people within their native *habitus*, as in the case of Amelia. The difference between women with broad capital and women with average capital lay not in their ability to reach out at least once, but in their ability to do so again and again, transforming initial encounters into ongoing bonds of mutual trust and support, the foundation from which social capital emerges.

Women with broad social capital demonstrated a wider exposure to people and groups different from themselves, including a broad range of middle-class professionals. They also demonstrated an enhanced ability to cross from one habitus to another. Women who fell closer to the "broad" end of the cultural-capital spectrum fell into several subgroups. Some reported work (Selma, Celestina, Nini) or educational histories (Nini, Caridad, Celestina) that exposed them to variants of a middle-class *habitus*. Others had long histories of institutionalization, exposing them to the norms of bureaucratic organizations and the professionals who run them (Nerina, Gabrielle). Most of these women also reported exposure to working-class or marginalized groups, often through time on the streets or recovery groups and programs (Julia, Gabrielle, Selma, Nerina, Deborah). Such broad exposure facilitates movement between one *habitus* and another, because it grants individuals familiarity with the cultural capital of each. While working with me, this same group of women consistently demonstrated a greater willingness to cross from one *habitus* to another to find the help they needed.

Women with average social capital demonstrated a marked preference for remaining within their own habitus, *and focusing on the friends, family, and neighborhood organizations that populated them.* Although women who fell closer to the "average" end of the cultural-capital spectrum emphasized their preference for staying within their own *habitus*, this meant different things for different women. For some, it literally meant staying at home (Juana, Amelia, Alicia). For others, it meant avoiding institutions and organizations that operated outside of their comfort zone (Cristina, Carlotta, Nilsa, Paquita) or limiting the number and scope of cross-*habitus* relationships they established (Flor, Luchita). But even women who preferred their own *habitus* could "stretch" under the right conditions and make important connections with gatekeepers and resource brokers outside of it (Luchita, Alicia, Flor, Juana). What they could not do was employ this as a consistent strategy for getting what they needed. If their initial attempts to find palatable help failed, they were more likely to withdraw into their own worlds and adopt a strategy of avoidance (see Bourgois 2003 for another example of this response).

*Just as women with average cultural capital could sometimes reach outside of their comfort zone for help, women with broad capital sometimes demonstrated gaps in their ability to solidify cross-*habitus *bonds.* Broad cultural capital lent women the ability to reach outside of their own *habitus* as part of a consistent strategy. It enhanced their ability to draw diverse individuals into their social networks. But it was no guarantee that this strategy would work every time. Gabrielle and Julia both struggled with the limits of their cultural capital. Gabrielle sometimes alienated clinic workers by being overly emotional, and Julia could not use middle-class strategies of organization and tracking because she had never learned them. However, women who had established a successful track record of boundary spanning were willing to make repeated attempts to cross outside of their *habitus* even though they sometimes floundered. They demonstrated an enhanced ability to adapt to new situations despite the risk.

In this small sample, women with average cultural capital were less likely to have a history of substance abuse, sex work, sexual abuse, or domestic violence;

they also reported fewer years of education and were less likely to be religiously observant. Women with broader cultural capital were more likely to be in recovery, report sexual abuse as either adults or children, and experience domestic violence. They were more likely to have been institutionalized, and they also reported more years of education. Most of those who reported some college education fell into this group. Finally, all of the eight women with broad cultural- and social-capital toolkits were religiously observant, as compared to four of the seven women with average toolkits.

Several of these patterns are striking. While it is not surprising that broader cultural and social capital was associated with higher levels of education, it is surprising that substance abuse and violence correlate with them as well. Berger's study of political participation among a group of HIV-positive women living in Detroit can shed light here. All reported histories of sex work and substance abuse, and most reported sexual or domestic abuse as well. This is a commonly noted pattern (Murphy 1991; Miller, Downs, and Testa 1993; Berger 2004). In my study, five of the seven women reporting substance abuse also reported sexual and/or domestic abuse. Berger, however, found a strong connection between political empowerment and the resources that women discovered through recovery programs.

> This chapter discusses the concept of life reconstruction as a process integral to the development of political empowerment for the respondents. It specifically focuses on the external resources discovered, cultivated, and used that created the conditions for internal resources to develop. During substance abuse treatment and recovery, for example, respondents were introduced to therapy, spirituality, the language of advocacy, advocacy education, and to city- and state-sponsored programs for HIV-positive women. After being exposed to some of the rudiments of advocacy, respondents adapted, expanded, and improved upon this foundation as they became active in their communities. . . . It is precisely in the ways the women extend themselves through their roles as workers, activists, advocates and helpers that create overlapping spheres of authority and networks that enlarge opportunities and possibilities. The ability to sustain ties with groups they are interested in while surviving a life-threatening disease allows for lasting connections to be made. (Berger 2004, 105, 185)

In other words, women in recovery programs were exposed to an entirely new *habitus* that offered new kinds of cultural capital from which social capital— and new forms of agency—could be built. Berger calls this the development of a "public voice." I argue that this kind of boundary spanning translates into greater health benefits and enhanced well-being for urban HIV-positive women. Often, cross-*habitus* bonds improved women's lives (Deborah, Nini, Nerina,

Selma, Caridad, Julia, Celestina). In some cases, they may even have lengthened them—remember the speed with which Alicia was introduced to her doctor and the manner in which Luchita found an advocate. It is likely that the ability to forge cross-*habitus* bonds is learned through experiences that broaden native cultural capital, allowing people to engage with others unlike themselves. In this way, broad cultural capital generates broad social capital, which can, in turn, be mined for survival-enhancing resources.

This analysis also suggests that while structural violence places crippling constraints on women's lives, it does not rob them of agency. Just as structure can limit agency through poverty and high levels of risk, it can also shape agency by exposing women to institutionalization, recovery programs, and diverse ethnic enclaves that invite them to broaden their native toolkits.

It is critical to note that although some women could "manage" the institutions they encountered better than others, this did not mean that those institutions were adequate or just. Neither survival nor quality of life should depend on boundary spanning. All of the women in this study faced the same SAVA-related problems: exposure to HIV and drug-related violence, lack of affordable housing, depression, burnout, and inadequate resources. They all deserved the same quality of care and the same access to resources. But those who could not forge cross-*habitus* bonds got minimal help and cursory care.

As I followed all of these women through a maze of clinics and services, I had ample opportunity to watch each one negotiate (or avoid negotiating) for medicine, money, and resources. But the organizations brokering access to these things had structural constraints of their own. Newark could only offer what little it had to give. The city's legacy of poverty and civil unrest had created a flourishing SAVA epidemic, and its political climate further facilitated the spread of HIV/AIDS. It took years for community-based organizations to find the funding and support they needed to help the city's HIV-positive women and men. By the time the women in my study began looking for help, Newark had just become a place capable of providing it.

3

Unpacking Newark's Epidemic

In order to understand the impact of cultural and social capital on the lives of Caridad and her cohorts, it is crucial to understand the city in which most of them lived. When I began planning my study in the mid-1990s, most of the women I worked with had just begun their journey as people living with HIV/AIDS. They moved within a national, regional, and municipal context that shaped what was possible. This chapter will offer a glimpse of the greater economic and political forces that shaped their worlds and framed their lives. It is far from comprehensive, because these stories could fill volumes. I have selected only what I deem to be critical, in the hopes that this will offer a greater context in which to understand Newark's resourceful women.

Snapshots of the HIV/AIDS epidemic across the nation and in four U.S. cities situate Newark's stories in the national and regional scene of the period. Each city offers parallels and contrasts to Newark; each one is also home to a vibrant Puerto Rican community. City sketches are drawn from a variety of sources, including the results of the 1999 National Rapid Assessment, Response, and Evaluation (RARE) initiative. The RARE initiative was established in response to a 1998 request from the Congressional Black Caucus of the United States that the secretary of the U.S. Department of Health and Human Services declare a public health emergency in the black communities impacted by HIV/AIDS (Needle et al. 2003). While not meant to be definitive or comprehensive, these sketches do convey both the omnipresence of SAVA and the constantly shifting nature of HIV/AIDS epidemics.

Women and HIV: The National Scene

In 1981, the CDC noticed an alarming increase in cases of Kaposi's sarcoma, a rare form of skin cancer (AIDS Education Global Information System n.d.). The *New York Times* ran an article announcing that doctors in New York and

California had diagnosed forty-one cases of the cancer, all appearing among homosexual men. Eight of the victims died less than twenty-four months after their diagnosis, and nine of these forty-one men developed severe defects in their immunological systems (Altman 1981).

The cancer was not thought to be contagious, but public health experts believed that precipitating conditions, such as viruses or environmental factors, might exist. "The best evidence against contagion," said one physician," is that no cases have been reported to date outside the homosexual community or in women" (Altman 1981). Early that year, scientists began referring to the mysterious condition as GRID (gay-related immune deficiency) but it was soon renamed AIDS (acquired immunodeficiency syndrome) (Johnson and Ross; LSU Law Center 1993). By the following year, 285 cases were reported in seventeen U.S. cities and five European countries. The CDC had discovered that both sexual contact and infected blood transmitted the disease. However, the underlying immune deficiencies seen in these AIDS cases was still unknown (Johnson and Ross).

In 1983, the CDC acknowledged that the female sex partners of men with AIDS were at risk of acquiring the virus (Kaiser Family Foundation Global HIV/AIDS Timeline). Nevertheless, HIV-positive women were largely overlooked until the mid-1980s. As late as 1991, it could still be said that to the extent women were considered at all, they were seen as carriers of the disease, not as people struggling to survive in their own right (LaGuardia 1991). By this time, the few studies that included women recruited sex workers and pregnant women to investigate transmission of the virus to male partners and fetuses (LaGuardia 1991, 21). But as early as 1986, some advocates and social scientists began to ask how HIV impacted women themselves.

During the early 1980s, qualitative research emerged as a useful tool in the arsenal against AIDS (Singer et al. 2001). These studies were framed by the urgent need to understand social and cultural facilitators of transmission. Some examined local culture's impact on drug use and sexual practices, which in turn affected women's risks and perceptions of risk (Worth 1986; Amaro 1988; Lewis and Waters 1988; Mays and Cochran 1988). This work helped to establish a qualitative approach to the study of HIV-positive women that emphasized the development of successful prevention strategies (Osmond et al. 1992; Alonso and Koreck 1993; Farmer, Good, and Lindenbaum 1993; Lewis 1993; Romero, Arguelles, and Rivero 1993; Romero 1993; Clatts 1994; de Zalduando and Bernard 1995). While many studies in this tradition examined the problems of HIV-positive women, their preventive focus made it difficult to centralize quality-of-life or care-related issues.

A smaller body of social science research focused on the everyday challenges facing HIV-positive women, especially women of color. Evelynn Hammonds's historical study examined the stereotyping of African American women with STDs, including HIV (Hammonds 1992). She addressed the history of mistrust between

African American communities and mainstream health care professionals, racist depictions of HIV-positive women of color in the media, and the stigma attached to HIV-positive women in the African American community itself (Thomas and Quinn 1991). Shortly afterward, Romero, Arguelles, and Rivero pointed out that HIV-positive Latina women were virtually invisible in the AIDS literature (Romero, Arguelles, and Rivero 1993, 347).

Health activists, health care professional advocates, cultural critics, and HIV-positive women themselves created most of the early literature about HIV-positive women's health and quality of life (Elisabeth 1987; Richardson 1988; Shayne and Kaplan 1991; Watstein and Laurich 1991; Bury, Morrison, and McLachlan 1992; Corea 1992; Dorn, Henderson, and South 1992; Henderson 1992; Douard and Durham 1993; Kneisl 1993; Kurth 1993; Weitz 1993; Patton 1994). They documented a long list of problems: poverty, lack of care, invisibility, gender roles that kept women from prioritizing their own needs, the absence of clinical research on women and HIV, and problems related to addiction. Most articles were case studies of individual women or general descriptions of the poor conditions they faced. Little information existed about the universe of treatments available to women or their impact on women's health, and studies about the use of complementary and alternative medicine (CAM) all focused on HIV-positive gay men (Whittaker 1991; Kurth 1993; Furin 1995).

Nineteen ninety-three and 1994 ushered in the HIV Epidemiology Research Study (HERS) and the Women's Interagency HIV Study (WIHS). Both were large, federally funded studies of women and HIV. The HERS study compared the health-service use and treatment regimens of HIV-positive and HIV-negative urban women. Although it found that almost 90 percent of HIV-positive women reported a usual and consistent source of care, almost 50 percent also reported a visit to the emergency room in the prior six months. Nearly 30 percent had not had a pelvic exam in the last year, and only 70 percent with CD4 counts below 500 had ever taken antiretroviral drugs (a normal CD4 count is between 500 and 1,400 cells/mm^3 of blood). Far more women had taken these medications than were currently using them. The study concluded that despite high levels of health care use, use of HIV-related services seemed inadequate (Solomon et al. 1998). The WIHS study followed a diverse group of HIV-positive and at-risk HIV-negative women, predominantly poor, urban women of color, over many years. The study was designed to explore the spectrum and course of HIV infection in women and the effects of treatment on them, providing multiple opportunities to improve their medical care (Barkan et al. 1998; Greenblatt et al. 1999). For example, it found that HIV-positive women were more likely to report genital-tract infections and symptoms than HIV-negative women, but fewer chlamydial and gonococcal infections (Greenblatt et al. 1999).

In 1994, the AIDS Clinical Trial Group 076 began testing the efficacy of AZT administered to HIV-positive mothers during pregnancy and to their children after birth as a method of preventing HIV transmission (Patterson 1994). The study showed that AZT lessened the likelihood of mother-to-child transmission by almost 68 percent, even though its long-term effects on both mother and child were unknown (Groves 1994; Patterson 1994; John and Kreiss 1996). These findings proved so compelling that the trial was stopped prematurely by officials at the National Institute of Allergy and Infectious Diseases, and all participating medical centers were told to offer AZT to pregnant women in the study who had been receiving a placebo (Patterson 1994).

Finally, in 1996, Highly Active Anti-Retroviral Therapy (HAART), a combination of three different classes of HIV medication, became available to people living with the virus in the Unites States. Almost immediately concerns were raised about equality of access to this new and ultimately life-extending treatment. Would it be equally available to current and former substance users, women and urban people of color? As I began planning my study and entering the field, such questions were as yet unresolved (Agins et al. 2004).

HIV/AIDS in the Midwest and Northeast:
The Regional Scene

Detroit

Detroit's early industrial success, the history of its automotive factories, and its postindustrial economic decline introduced it into the national imagination (Herron 1993; Berger 2004). Michele Berger's analysis of the political development of a group of inner city HIV-positive women offers a brief glimpse into this city's HIV/AIDS epidemic. The women in her sample bore a striking resemblance to Newark's resourceful women, despite the fact that most identified as African American and all reported a history of drug use. The women who worked with Berger grappled with poverty, stigma, compromised access to health care, high rates of exposure to personal and familial drug abuse, sexual assault, and limited opportunities for themselves and their children. All were exposed to high-risk activities throughout their lives, and all contracted the virus either directly or indirectly through the drug trade (Berger 2004). Like Newark, Detroit's HIV/AIDS epidemic is serious compared to its surrounding area, and the city was slow to respond to the HIV/AIDS virus. Also like Newark, city residents experienced extreme isolation and poverty throughout the eighties (Herron 1993; Berger 2004). HIV-positive women living in Detroit (and in Michigan) were often assumed by clinical and social service workers to be addicts and sex workers,, and legislators passed punitive laws targeting those with children and those who became pregnant (Berger 2004).

Detroit has long grappled with ethnic balkanization, and its many communities of color have struggled to access the city's limited resources. The public school system suffered as residents left the city to settle into self-contained economic systems based in surrounding communities. Like Newark, Detroit has yet to recover from the devastation following its 1967 riots (Bergmann 2008).

In the tumult of the late sixties and early seventies, southwest Detroit's Latino communities banded together with the Michigan Department of Public Health, the Michigan Department of Social Services, and the Detroit Health Department to establish the Community Health and Social Services Center (CHASS). It began providing limited medical services to the Mexican and Puerto Rican communities from a renovated house on a main thoroughfare. As demand for low-cost and no-cost medical care increased, CHASS expanded to become the primary source of health care for Spanish-speaking residents (CHASS). In 1971, two local community-based organizations (the Latino Mental Health Task Force and La Casa) combined to become Latino Family Services. When the HIV/AIDS epidemic emerged in Detroit, CHASS (now a federally qualified health center, or FQHC) and Latino Family Services were positioned to provide culturally sensitive HIV/AIDS prevention services and clinical care to the area's Mexican and Puerto Rican communities (Latino Family Services n.d.).

Chicago

Chicago suffered from the decline of the postwar industrial boom, which led to the closing of factories, steel mills, stockyards, and other industries along the city's South Side. The steady loss of jobs hit the city's working-class African Americans especially hard, although all local communities of color also suffered. During the 1980s, AIDS cases appeared most frequently among men who had sex with other men (MSMs). Most were non-Latino whites. But over time, both the primary mode of transmission and the most vulnerable populations changed, as later cases were directly or indirectly linked to drug injection. For many years, African American communities have reported the greatest number of cases, although the city's Puerto Rican and white communities have also faced elevated risks. The incidence of HIV/AIDS has steadily increased in the city's women of color over time (LaKosky, Ward, and Ouellet 2007).

RARE researchers in Chicago found that trends in injection drug use varied widely by race/ethnicity and community area at the time of their study: they noted that most African American injection drug users (IDUs) were over thirty, while white IDUs were identified across many age groups. Some neighborhoods had limited access to needle-exchange programs; others had more, but funding restrictions limited what they could do. In each neighborhood investigated, the epidemic took on a slightly different form (LaKosky, Ward, and Ouellet 2007).

When the HIV/AIDS crisis emerged in Chicago's West Town Puerto Rican community, a group of activists and community members decided to organize. "Instead of importing and accommodating models based on middle-class gay, Anglo sensibilities—gay, bisexual, and straight Latino community activists cobbled together a few resources and in 1998 created Vida/SIDA" (Sanabria 2004, 37).

This community-based, organically generated organization offered culturally appropriate HIV prevention, education, and treatment services to Chicago's Puerto Rican residents. "In its infancy, Vida/SIDA, which translates as Life/AIDS, was solely an alternative health clinic for people with AIDS. Free of charge, it provided services such as acupuncture, massage therapy, chiropractic care, nutritional counseling, and even t'ai chi" (Sanabria 2004, 37).

At first, Vida/SIDA operated out of a law firm's office after hours. It tailored its services to the needs of local residents, including the communities' many single mothers and the wives of HIV-positive MSM. By 2004, Vida/SIDA occupied two locations: one dedicated to education outreach and another treating HIV-positive community residents. In part because of Vida/SIDA's efforts, HIV/AIDS case rates among Puerto Ricans declined steadily in Chicago, showing that a community that organized its cultural and social capital could help turn around the spread of this syndemic (Sanabria 2004).

Hartford

Hartford is situated in one of the wealthiest U.S. states, but it is one of only four that saw an increase in the rate of poverty between 1990 and 2000 (Connecticut Department of Public Health 2002). Nearly 60 percent of families with children are headed by single women, and more teenage girls give birth than graduate from high school. Poverty and unemployment levels are high. In 2000, 48 percent of the babies born were Latino or African American.

As in other impoverished U.S. cities, HIV/AIDS in Hartford is linked to injection drug use, commercial sex, and high-risk sexual activity among MSM. However, Hartford's noninjecting drug users have far higher than average levels of HIV infection. RARE researchers in this city also found that most of the individuals they interviewed fell into two or more risk categories at the same time. Crack cocaine users in Hartford were at very high risk of HIV infection because over half also injected heroin and most were sex workers. The Hartford RARE team recommended that late-night outreach, syringe exchange, and prevention services be created, since most risky behavior took place at night, when agencies were closed. It also recommended the immediate creation of an all-night, safe drop-in center for women and, eventually, a similar one for men (Singer and Eiserman 2007).

Despite these challenges, Hartford has a powerful advantage in addressing the city's poverty, drug, and AIDS crisis. For over twenty years, the Hispanic Health Council (HHC) and its daughter organization, the Institute for Community Research (ICR) have provided an interdisciplinary, community-based approach to the development, implementation, management, and evaluation of HIV-prevention projects. They have targeted high-risk populations, especially drug users, sex partners of drug users, commercial sex workers, adolescents, farm workers, and gay men and youth (Singer and Weeks 2005).

In doing so, the HHC and ICR have generated their own model of community-based HIV/AIDS research.

> The roots of the Hartford Model, which are embedded most deeply in Action and Advocacy Anthropology . . . date to the end of the Second World War, long before the founding of either the Hispanic Health Council or the Institute for Community Research. . . . Application of the model began in the late 1970s with community efforts to address pressing health problems in the burgeoning Puerto Rican population. Attracted by available work in the nearby tobacco fields, Puerto Ricans had begun migrating to Hartford in growing numbers during the 1960s. In their new home, Puerto Ricans—a group that has had American citizenship since the First World War—faced the triple burden of poverty, discrimination, and cultural and linguistic difference from the dominant population. Health and other social institutions were ill prepared to respond to the needs of this growing community and, as a result, were not particularly inclined initially to become more responsive. Reacting to this mainstream indifference, a core of Puerto Rican community health activists developed and soon found willing partners among a small group of applied anthropologists affiliated with the University of Connecticut. (Singer and Weeks 2005, 157–158)

When the AIDS epidemic emerged in Hartford around 1987, activist researchers at the HHC and ICR applied the model to issues of drug- and sex-related HIV risk, eventually introducing the concept of the SAVA syndemic (Singer 1994; Singer 1996; Baer, Singer, and Susser 1997). By combining the characteristics of a community-based service organization with an academic research institute, the HHC and ICR were able to offer a roster of services to both the Latino and African American community, including culturally sensitive, gender-specific drug-treatment and AIDS-prevention programs. The HHC and ICR have also partnered with other community health and service organizations in Hartford to conduct an AIDS-prevention demonstration project and develop culturally targeted intervention programs for drug users and their sex partners living in predominantly Puerto Rican and African American parts of the city (Singer and Weeks 2005).

New York

The national impact of New York City's HIV/AIDS epidemic is better addressed by a book than a sketch. Fortunately, Susan Chambré's volume *Fighting for Our Lives* takes on the social history of the AIDS community in New York City, introducing its epic proportions in this way:

> Far from a typical American city, New York has been the center of the epidemic in the United States, and a place where many organizational

models and policies were created. The city was hit early and hit hard by the epidemic. Half of the reported cases in the nation before 1983 were in New York. By the early 1990s, the disease was the third major cause of death for men in the city, and the fifth for women. Its effect was so enormous that it actually played an important role in reducing, between 1983 and 1992, life expectancy at birth for white men in the city by 1.1 years. In 1993, New York City had more cases than the next forty cities combined, and individual neighborhoods had more cases than many states. In 2001, New York City's AIDS case rate of 65.9 per 100,000 people was nearly double San Francisco's (34.6), six times the rate in Boston (10.8), and four times the U.S. average (14.9). A total of 128,141 people in New York City were diagnosed with AIDS in the United States during the first two decades of the epidemic. . . . New York's AIDS community emerged early . . . [and] included the largest number, and most specialized, of formal and informal AIDS organizations in the nation. New York–based organizations were often the first of their type, like the Gay Men's Health Crisis (GMHC), the first AIDS organization in the world. New York was also the birthplace of the AIDS Coalition to Unleash Power, ACT UP, probably the best known advocacy organization. . . . Many served as models for groups in the United States and throughout the world . . . and benefited from the private funding available from foundations, corporations, and new AIDS charities located in the city. Many also relied heavily on funds from New York State's AIDS Institute. (Chambré 2006, 4–5)

Chambré focuses on the pivotal role of gay men in the early years of the epidemic. She describes the role of the PWA (People with AIDS) Coalition in emphasizing individual and community empowerment. She notes that GMHC generated the earliest models of HIV/AIDS support and service provision. Chambré also describes key contributions by elite women and faith-community leaders, making it clear that the city's epidemic was met by a powerful coalition of individuals with broad cultural and social capital. She also points out that this kind of massive mobilization occurred much later in New York City's communities of color and among its injection drug users, partly due to "limited economic and social capital in these communities" (Chambré 2006, 8). The gap in capital between the city's disparate communities mirrors that between New York and Newark.

However, members of New York's Puerto Rican community played active roles in the city's fight against AIDS. One such individual was Yolanda Serrano, a Puerto Rican community worker who became the president of ADAPT, the Association of Drug Abuse Prevention and Treatment. This organization created a model of AIDS outreach to IDUs by sending volunteers into shooting galleries to counsel drug users about how to avoid HIV. The group was the first to develop and distribute bleach kits for cleaning needles and syringes. Serrano is probably best known for forcing New York State to sponsor a needle-exchange pilot program after it rejected the city's request to do so in May of 1987. "Without the backing of ADAPT's board, Serrano told a *New York Times* reporter that the agency was willing to break the law and distribute clean needles and collect used ones. The front-page story indicated that they were willing to risk their funding and tax exemption" to do so (Chambré 2006, 164). Eventually, this move had its intended effect: it reopened public conversation about needle exchange and caused the governor to approve the pilot, making it the second legal needle exchange in the country and the first operated by a city government (Chambré 2006). While this proved to be only the beginning of a long struggle to legalize needle exchange, and eventually the sale of needles to the public, it was a critical first step.

Newark

Newark's poverty cannot be solely attributed to the 1967 conflict known alternately as "the riots" or "the rebellion," but the five days of destruction shaped the nature of its impoverishment (Hayden 1967; Herman 2007; NPR 2007; King 2007; Mumford 2007; Parks 2007a; Parks 2007b; Parks 2007c; Porambo, Sloat, and Bruning 2007). Twenty-six persons died, countless numbers were wounded and the crisis made a lasting impression on the national consciousness. Eugenia Lee Hancock observes that "Newark's past appears to be stuck in 1967. . . . Newark has a stain upon it, its identity forever mediated by the ever present memory of riots, destruction, looting, and mayhem" (Hancock 2002, 57). Activist and attorney Junius Williams has described the event as a "riot within a rebellion" in which unarmed citizens protested joblessness, racist Federal Housing Authority policies, dilapidated housing, poor public health, and "geographic apartheid" through demonstrations and looting (Hayden 1967; King 1987; Hancock 2002; Herman 2007; King 2007; Mumford 2007; Parks 2007a). Panicking authorities and inexperienced National Guardsmen responded with bullets (Herman 2005; NPR 2007; Parks 2007a; Parks 2007b; Parks 2007c; Porambo, Sloat, and Bruning 2007). Official inquiries into potential police wrongdoing resulted in no indictments, creating scars that persist to this day (King 2007).

From 1970 to 1975, Newark lost forty-two thousand citizens, as whites and middle-class blacks left in search of new job opportunities and a safer, more pleasant place to live. They took their tax dollars with them, leaving behind a crumbling infrastructure with an inadequate tax base. To make matters worse, 76 percent of the municipality's most valuable properties were granted tax-exempt status and could not be tapped for cash (Hancock 2002).

The illegal drug industry expanded in the economic vacuum created by lost jobs and wealth. Easy access to IV drugs led to an explosion of addicts living in the city, creating a perfect environment for the spread of HIV (Thomas 1993). The popularity of "shooting galleries"—abandoned buildings where needles could be rented and shared—added to the problem (Whitlow 1986e; Whitlow 1991). This combination promoted the spread of HIV/AIDS in Newark, spearheading a heterosexual epidemic among male IV drug injectors and their female partners.

By 1990, Newark's home county of Essex had the highest number of AIDS cases in the state. It was the only New Jersey county with more than fifty cases per hundred thousand (Leusner 1990b). By 1998, when New York, San Francisco, and Miami had all reduced their rates of reported AIDS cases, Newark had gotten worse, going from 44.6 percent to 47 percent that same year (Curtis et al. 2007). The city's economic condition did not improve during this period either: in 1993, Newark became the eleventh poorest city in the United States. Almost seventy-one thousand of its residents, or 26 percent of the population, lived below the poverty line (Thomas 1993).

Newark's impoverished residents responded to the HIV/AIDS epidemic very differently than New York's gay white community. Few of the city's HIV-positive residents were "the extraordinarily privileged and well connected people" who were falling ill in other parts of the country (Hancock 2002, 67). Though small and medium-sized grassroots organizations emerged early on to answer the challenge, their members had neither the economic nor political clout required to create a solid infrastructure for the city's PWAs. Instead, these CBOs (community-based organizations) fought to survive on volunteer labor and small grants that appeared infrequently if at all. "Due to the poverty and political disenfranchisement of [Newark's] gay community and the invisibility of women and drug users, AIDS remained unnamed, unrecognized, unnoticed, and untreated far longer in Newark than in the city eleven miles away [New York City]" (Hancock 2002, 68).

Newark's RARE research team reported a high frequency of multidrug use in the city. Injection equipment, difficult to access in the absence of needle-exchange programs, was hoarded and reused again and again, increasing the risk of HIV infection. Hard drug use was noted as a serious problem for both the city's African American and Puerto Rican communities. Despite considerable HIV-related funding, the team also found an "alarming lack of visible or effective [HIV] outreach being done in the city. . . . There was no apparent evidence of outreach activities of any kind. . . . When asked, people had never seen outreach conducted in their neighborhoods." On a more promising note, RARE's final report had a strong impact on agency outreach programs, increasing their scope and frequency and improving the way services were provided. The team's findings were also used by primary care clinics to alter the hours when services were offered. Finally, dedicated clinics serving gay and transgendered individuals were established in response to the report's findings (Curtis et al. 2007).

Newark Stories

Four of Newark's stories tell us something valuable about our nation's AIDS epidemic. The first is the story of HIV-positive women, who were overlooked for years after AIDS arrived in the city. The second explores the pivotal but under-recognized role of the Puerto Rican community in the fight against the virus. The third story follows city officials who denied what was happening: by attempting to shield their constituents from the threat of AIDS, they sacrificed those who fell victim to it. The last story is about the role of cultural and social capital in shaping the epidemic. All have been reconstructed from four decades of newspaper stories, journals, film documentaries, and radio interviews.

State and city officials were slow to recognize that AIDS was a heterosexual problem in Newark and even slower to act on the risk it posed for women. In 1978, a five-year-old girl was admitted to Newark's Beth Israel Medical Hospital. Known as Patient 6, she suffered from an unknown illness. The child was put under the care of pediatrician Dr. James Oleske. Despite the efforts of the pediatric team, she died (Underdue 1991; Campbell 2006). Oleske could not explain what was happening, but he saved a sample of her blood that later proved she had died of AIDS. Later, he would come to believe that hers was the first documented case of AIDS in the world (Campbell 2006). It is probable, though not certain, that Patient 6 contracted HIV in utero from her mother, who acquired it either through sex with an IV drug user or IV drug use herself. Newark's first known casualty of the HIV/AIDS epidemic was neither a gay man nor an addict, but a child whose illness mirrored that of her mother.

When the New Jersey Department of Health began tracking AIDS cases in 1983 no category existed for heterosexual victims of the disease (Whitlow 1987b). By 1984, the New Jersey State Department of Health reported that AIDS had killed 127 New Jersey residents since the disease had been officially recognized in 1981. "The majority of cases occur among IV drug users and homosexuals, according to experts," noted an article in the *Star-Ledger* (Whitlow 1984). Despite this, New Jersey's Department of Health started tracking a new category of AIDS cases: "sexual partners of a member of an at-risk group." By mid-March, three women made up this category (Whitlow 1987b).

Even this early, the Newark metropolitan area was taking the lead in numbers of AIDS cases. Officials already knew that 46 percent of city residents diagnosed with the illness had contracted it from IV drug use; it was also clear that this was different from the pattern emerging in the rest of the country. There, most of the ill were members of the gay male community (Schulte 1985a). In Newark, however, two-thirds were heterosexual IV drug users (Schulte 1985b).

By 1987 Health Commissioner Coye and other state officials had focused on IV drug use. Coye asserted that the only way to stop AIDS in New Jersey was to stop drug abuse, since 60 percent of the state's cases resulted directly or indirectly from it (Peet and Whitlow 1987). This simple formula discouraged the state from focusing on the insidious relationship between IV drug addiction, gender relations, and the rise of HIV among women.

Community workers and front-line doctors like James Oleske understood that many HIV-positive women were not IV drug users themselves, but had partnered with them. Half did not even know their husbands or boyfriends were addicts before giving birth to HIV-positive babies (Peet and Whitlow 1987; Campbell 2006). Sadly, these facts could not compete with a more sensational way of framing the problem.

The December 20, 1987, issue of Newark's *Star-Ledger* featured the first of a three-part series about Newark's HIV-positive children. It was called "Kids with AIDS: Jersey Struggles with a 'Deadly Legacy.'" The series introduced readers to the growing number of HIV-positive children in the city. It was also one of the first widely read pieces to focus on HIV-positive women. It told the painful stories of children adrift in the foster care system and the drug-addicted women who had abandoned them; Oleske's insights about the wives and girlfriends of IV drug users were compressed into two sentences at the end of the first article (Peet 1987a).

The first installment told readers about Cynthia, a two-and-a-half-year-old HIV-positive baby. It was accompanied by a picture of a beautiful little girl smiling at the camera. The story described the city's HIV-positive women in the worst possible terms:

New Jersey has the highest percent of women AIDS victims in their child bearing years of any state. . . . Many are unaware that they carry the disease. Pitifully few have made the behavioral changes necessary to save the children. . . . The infected children—innocent victims in the most profound sense—will all die. . . . The epidemic has also created a generation of 'boarder babies,' newborns abandoned because their mothers are dead or dying themselves or otherwise incapable of raising them. (Peet 1987a)

Cynthia's foster mother estimated that Newark was home to between ten thousand and fifteen thousand of the latter, a group of "hardcore female addicts, the majority of which support their habit by prostitution."

The series downplayed several important facts and omitted others. It brushed over the large number of women who never knew that their husbands and boyfriends had a history of using drugs. It did not encourage women to ask themselves if they might be at risk, nor did it question why so few community-based drug treatment programs were accessible to women. The series did not report the greatly accelerated death rates of women diagnosed with AIDS. Instead of telling readers that their average time from diagnosis to death was less than four months—far less than the national average of eighteen months—the *Star-Ledger* series painted Newark's HIV-positive women as child abusers, prostitutes, and unrepentant IV drug addicts (Peet 1987a; Peet 1987b; Peet 1987c).

In doing so, the series both reflected and helped shape a larger national trend, described in Gena Corea's book *The Invisible Epidemic: The Story of Women and AIDS* (1992). When women were first recognized in the context of the epidemic, they were seen as disease carriers, not potential victims (LaGuardia 1991; Corea 1992); national attention focused on sex workers and pregnant women, as politicians and researchers worried about transmission to men and fetuses. The *Star-Ledger* series would be a part of this larger trend, painting a picture that would linger locally for decades to come.

Sixteen days after the series ended, the city council passed an ordinance requiring that anyone arrested for prostitution be tested for AIDS (Narvaez 1988). Police began arresting sex workers and their customers along South Broad Street. Mayor Sharpe James first vetoed the law and then refused to enforce it, saying it was unconstitutional (Byrd 1988a). Gay advocacy groups were fiercely against it, but representatives from other states began calling Newark officials to ask for information so they could propose similar laws. A South Carolina official explained why: "We want to track these people and see if they are spreading AIDS" (Byrd 1988a). What he meant was that they wanted to track female sex workers to see if they posed a danger to the men who used their services as well as to their own infants.

In late 1988, University Hospital (UMDNJ) received both a $4.8 million dollar grant to study the vertical (mother-to-child) transmission of HIV and a $13.8 million dollar grant—its largest ever—to study heterosexual transmission of the disease (Whitlow 1988e; Whitlow 1988d). The first study would focus on Newark, while the second would be conducted in three cities: Newark, Paterson, and Jersey City. The vertical transmission study, in particular, would make an experimental treatment available to a group of HIV-positive pregnant women who would not have had access to it otherwise. But Newark's female PWAs probably attracted the attention of funding institutions not because of their need, but because they were part of a "natural experiment," and the city's heterosexual epidemic made a vertical transmission study possible. To be fair, James Oleske pointed out that grant money meant more nurses, technicians, and doctors to provide AIDS care. It also created the opportunity to offer improved counseling, diagnosis, and assessments. "It is not just a matter of wanting money and permission to use people as guinea pigs" (Whitlow 1986b).

Some of Newark's women did find themselves receiving better care. Nineteen eighty-eight also saw the creation of the first AIDS clinic exclusively for women. This University Hospital clinic had a caseload of three hundred and made do with only five doctors. There was a long waiting list for new clients, but the clinic's impact on the health of its patients was profound. The period from diagnosis to death among patients enrolled there would go from 14.5 weeks in 1988 to 70 weeks in 1989, compared to a lengthening of only 24 weeks for New Jersey women who didn't get help (Leusner 1990a).

The clinic was the first to use full-time social workers, and it began making sure that all patients were connected to the full range of services for which they were eligible. Under the direction of Dr. Patricia Kloser it continued to expand modestly until it served over five hundred women. If more money had been available, Kloser said she could have handled twice that many: "I would like to advertise what I do here, but I'm afraid to. I don't want to be turning people away, but we are already way overbooked" (McLaughlin 1992a).

The New Jersey Women and AIDS Network (NJWAN), a nonprofit, grassroots organization, was founded in the same year as the women's clinic. It would remain the only "female-specific AIDS service organization in the state" and be among the first nationally to focus on HIV-infected and -affected women. NJWAN began advocating for women all over the state, pushing for policies to support them and creating programs to educate service providers and health care professionals about their needs. One of its central missions was to empower women affected by the virus, encouraging them to help each other and advocate for themselves (NJWAN). NJWAN would play a crucial role in directing resources toward New Jersey women coping with HIV/AIDS throughout the epidemic.

In 1989 New Jersey Health Commissioner Dr. Molly Joel Coye announced that one in two hundred babies born in New Jersey carried the AIDS virus. A CDC-funded study released these findings after testing the blood of virtually all babies born during a three-month period (Schwaneberg 1989). At University Hospital (UMDNJ) in Newark, one in twenty-two infants tested positive for HIV antibodies (Wyckoff 1989). It became clear that the virus was reaching greater numbers of New Jersey women than had been previously imagined.

Shortly after, public perceptions of women living with HIV/AIDS showed evidence of change. A September 1990 story in the *Star-Ledger* featured a woman named Karen Ann, a thirty-two-year-old single parent who had acquired HIV from a partner. Her story represented a radical departure from media depictions of HIV-positive women who used drugs and abandoned their children. Karen was described as a responsible working mother who lost her thirty-thousand-dollar-a-year job because of her illness (Stewart 1990). Two weeks later, the *Star-Ledger* reported that heterosexuals who did not use intravenous drugs had become the fastest growing group of people to acquire AIDS in New Jersey. One in nine AIDS cases diagnosed in the previous year had been in people who contracted the disease through heterosexual contact rather than direct drug use, representing an increase of 185 percent over the preceding year (Leusner 1990b).

On December 1, 1990—World AIDS Day—New Jersey's new health commissioner, Frances Dunston, delivered a major address on the topic of AIDS, saying that too little attention had been paid to the "special medical and social needs of women" (Aun 1990). Appropriately enough, that year's World AIDS Day theme was "Women and AIDS." Dunston focused on the need to expand drug treatment for women, but Sandra Elkin, a film producer speaking at the same event, took an entirely different view of the matter. "We have not been provided with realistic tools that will help us be protected from infection," she argued. "We began, very early in this epidemic, to leave out the important messages for women. We gave women half the story. We told women to ask their partners [about their sexual or drug abuse history] but we left out some important information: men lie to women" (Aun 1990). Elkin went on to cite a study showing that 35 percent of men surveyed said that they did not tell their women partners the truth about their sexual and drug histories.

At University Hospital (UMDNJ), the new clinical trial targeting pregnant women had just begun. Patricia Kloser, director of the Newark Women's AIDS Clinic, had begun referring her pregnant patients to Dr. Arlene Bardequez, an OB/GYN professor at UMDNJ. Bardequez was directing what would become known as the "076" trial, which would test the efficacy of AZT administered to HIV-positive mothers during pregnancy and to their child after birth as a method of preventing the transmission of HIV (Patterson 1994). This study, which AIDS researchers commonly refer to as "076," was such a watershed in AIDS research that it remains well known to this day.

The trial was controversial because the effects of AZT on both the fetus and the mother were unknown. In order to qualify for the study, women were required to have relatively healthy immune systems because AZT might seriously lower their current levels of immunity or harm their unborn babies. Thus, the decision to participate was a risky one, but doing nothing might mean that a baby would grow up HIV-positive. Kloser explained that "A lot of women, for religious and other reasons, have no choice but to carry [their fetuses]. It's a scary thought in terms of guilt—if they give birth to a positive baby—and the work involved, which could compromise their own health . . . so these women who . . . enroll[ed] at the time were very brave, because of the controversy and the unknown" (Patterson 1994).

Kloser's patients ranged in age from seventeen to seventy-seven, but most were between thirty and thirty-nine. Ninety percent were pregnant or were already mothers. Half had contracted the disease from sex with an infected partner. Describing her clients, Kloser said: "I love my patients. Most of them are young. They are sick. They have lots of strikes against them in their lives even without AIDS. They come here and sometimes they wait for hours. Sometimes they have to leave without seeing me because they have children at home that need attention or because the man they are living with is too sick and needs their help. They always put their children first. I admire them, really. I wish I had their courage" (McLaughlin 1992a).

Increasingly, the needs of women were becoming more and more visible and small, local CBOs began providing them with services and support. Organizations like Northern Lights Alternatives offered everything from workshops on coping—the AIDS Mastery Workshop—to children's clothes and sofas (Patterson 1993). Slowly, larger organizations began to follow suit. The New Jersey AIDS Partnership awarded one hundred thousand dollars to six Newark area community service programs and grants of up to fifty thousand dollars for the training of public policy advocates for HIV-positive women affected by the disease (*Star-Ledger* 1993). Grantees included the United Hospitals of Newark's Family Place, offering outreach and home care for women and their families, the Women's Rights Litigation Clinic of Rutgers Law School, NJWAN, and Vivian's Place, a holistic health resource center, lounge, and workshop for HIV-positive women sponsored by the AIDS Interfaith Network (*Star-Ledger* 1993; Wyckoff 1993).

The new emphasis on HIV/AIDS services for women had not come soon enough—AIDS was now the leading killer of women aged twenty-five to forty-four in Newark. Most of the city's HIV-positive women were African American or Hispanic—primarily Puerto Rican. The clear majority were the wives and girlfriends of HIV-positive drug users (Thomas 1993). Dr. Anita Vaughn, medical director of the Newark Community Center on Ludlow Street, spoke to Jerry Thomas, a staff writer at the *Chicago Tribune*, about the way in which Newark's women were affected by the epidemic. As one of the city's most experienced AIDS care physicians, she was intimately familiar with the situation. Her health care center provided treatment services to women and their families, helped patients write out wills, assisted in decision making about the future care of children, and helped locate foster homes when necessary. They also hosted a weekly support group for women with AIDS. The clinic, located in the Dayton Street Projects, witnessed the poverty and addiction fueling the epidemic on a day-to-day basis. "The women say they survive by adopting a healthier lifestyle and by blocking out negative thoughts," explained Dr. Vaughn (Thomas 1993).

A breakthrough for the treatment of HIV-positive women and their infants emerged when researchers at the 076 trial found that only 8 percent of the babies of mothers receiving AZT contracted HIV, while 26 percent of the placebo babies became infected (Patterson 1994). These findings proved so compelling that the trial was stopped prematurely by officials at the National Institute of Allergy and Infectious Diseases. All participating medical centers were told to offer AZT to pregnant women in the study who had been receiving a placebo

(Patterson 1994). By April, Governor Christie Whitman was urging all pregnant women to take an AIDS test and consider the use of AZT if their tests were positive (Groves 1994). But others were more cautious.

Marion Banzhaf, NJWAN's director, asked for an independent review of the findings; she raised concerns about future side effects of the drug and pointed out that adverse effects of treatment would only be apparent at the end of a full study (Groves 1994). Until then, any potential long-term side effects would remain unknown. Despite her concerns and those of others in the HIV community, physicians and researchers embraced the 076 results. The standard of care for HIV-positive pregnant women was quickly modified to include the administration of AZT to the mother during pregnancy and labor, and to the infant for several weeks after birth.

By August 1995 an updated needs assessment report noted that the previous year had seen an increase of 2,894 HIV/AIDS cases in the region around Newark and that women now accounted for 31 percent of all cases, more than double the national average of 14 percent. Of all HIV-positive women in the region, 81 percent were black, 11 percent were white, and 7.6 percent were Hispanic (Soto 1995). The epidemic was exploding among urban women of color. Yet even this late, Nick Macchione, executive director of the Newark HIV Planning Council, said that the number of HIV-positive women in the area was "alarming and puzzling," adding that researchers were unable to explain why it was so high.

As a member of the state HIV Prevention Community Planning Group, he was part of the team tackling the issue. "We still don't have a finger on the pulse," he explained. "These women are spouses of injecting drug users (IDUs). Because the number of IDU cases is increasing, so is the number of women [with HIV or AIDS]" (Soto 1995). Unbelievably, after more than a decade of living with Newark's SAVA syndemic, city officials still fumbled in the face of its threat to women.

Newark's Puerto Rican community often went unrecognized for its role in confronting the AIDS epidemic. In the Spanish-speaking community, CBOs like CURA and FOCUS worked quietly on behalf of Newark's Hispanics; PROCEED did the same for residents of Elizabeth, Newark's sister city. CURA specialized in offering drug treatment to local Puerto Ricans and Hispanics. In 1978, it began to experience a noticeable surge in demand for its services. An unidentified illness was moving through its clients, most of whom were current or prior IV drug users. The organization geared up to meet the new challenge, widening its outreach (CURA). When the CBO was given the opportunity to learn more by participating in a CDC study, they jumped at the chance. CURA collected blood samples from residential drug treatment clients who agreed to participate and forwarded them to the CDC. Clients were reimbursed, but the agency received no payment. This was the beginning of CURA's HIV/AIDS program (CURA).

As the epidemic progressed, attention focused on CBOs and grassroots organizations working on behalf of the city's PWAs. A 1988 article in the *Star-Ledger* highlighted the most active AIDS organizations in New Jersey and the greater Newark area. It profiled New Jersey Buddies, the Gay Activist Alliance of New Jersey, New Brunswick's Hyacinth Foundation, New Jersey ACT UP, and the PWA Coalition, as well as drug rehabilitation centers like Soul-O-House and Integrity House. In the article, Soul-O-House director Edna Thomas explained the pressing need for HIV/AIDS resources designed for the city's black communities (Whitlow 1988c).

However, there was no mention of Newark's large Puerto Rican and Hispanic communities, nor was CURA profiled, despite years of AIDS-related work (Whitlow 1988c). As Newark journalist Frederick W. Byrd observed, the city's flourishing Puerto Rican community remained strangely "invisible" to Newark's government and business sectors, including the media, despite its vibrant presence and many active organizations (Byrd 1983). As part of this trend, CURA, PROCEED, and the Latinos they served were virtually ignored outside of the Hispanic- and AIDS-service communities.

Yet grassroots organizations like CURA remained highly active throughout the epidemic despite a lack of reliable funding. They depended on volunteers or minimum-wage outreach workers to do community outreach, condom distribution, and promotion of confidential HIV testing. Many of these workers came from Newark's Puerto Rican community (Wyckoff 1993). Their bilingual, bicultural backgrounds positioned them perfectly to help their Spanish-speaking neighbors.

Two such advocate-workers were profiled in a 1992 *Star-Ledger* article. Liz Charriez and Irma Vasquez conducted outreach for the Essex Treatment Center in neighborhoods characterized by high rates of violent crime, drug use, and prostitution. They communicated with up to 150 people during a typical day and arranged to test up to five, a small but significant number (McLaughlin 1992b). At the best of times, organizations like theirs operated under severe financial constraints. The Essex Treatment Center paid only $16,500 a year for Charriez's full-time work and $8.50 an hour for Vasquez's part-time efforts. Care was taken to conserve money whenever possible; workers even retraced their steps to retrieve discarded pamphlets for reuse (McLaughlin 1992b).

Larger organizations like the Red Cross could count on a little more funding. Charriez eventually moved from the Essex Treatment Center to the Red Cross to take advantage of a pay increase (McLaughlin 1992b). The Red Cross was also able to find the funds for a mobile testing unit that stopped regularly at public housing complexes, welfare hotels, and other locations serving low-income, minority individuals (Whitlow 1992). The van was crucial for reaching women and children without easy access to HIV testing and retesting. Outreach workers noted that many of the male HIV-positive IV drug users they met showed little interest in preventing transmission of the virus. One outreach worker was quoted as saying, "They don't care. . . . They say, 'don't give me nothing and don't give my girl nothing either'" (Whitlow 1992). Without the presence of vans and bilingual workers, many women would have missed the opportunity to get tested and find help.

But not all of the city's Latino residents supported HIV/AIDS work so whole-heartedly. When Newark's zoning board allowed the AIDS consortium to lease part of a nursing home in 1993, the decision distressed the local Spanish-speaking community. The consortium had planned to establish a long-term care facility for AIDS patients, but the neighborhood refused to allow it. Despite ten years of HIV/AIDS education, the stigma of AIDS was too powerful. "Spokesmen for a group of Hispanic residents who live near the nursing home had maintained the project would be 'detrimental' to the neighborhood," reported the *Star-Ledger*. At a hearing designed to explore the problem, residents rejected the testimony of three experts denying that there would be any risk to locals; they were unmoved by the fact that 14 percent of New Jersey's PWAs were Hispanic and the facility would be serving members of their own ethnic community (Kukla 1993).

Armando Aviles, the lead spokesman for the group, cross-examined the experts and concluded that "There are too many unanswered questions about AIDS to locate this facility in such a densely populated area" (Kukla 1993). He raised concerns about the disposal of medical waste, the possible dangers of HIV transmission, and the proximity of the facility to two schools, including a future elementary school (Kukla 1993). Neighborhood residents also expressed the fear that people with AIDS would be walking neighborhood streets or standing in long lines in front of the facility (Whitlow 1994).

A UMDNJ administrator pointed out that the facility would have its own entranceway, two full-time security guards, and separate, self-contained heating and air conditioning units. Commissioner Daniel Webster, representing the majority vote, noted that "There's AIDS all around us. We're not bringing any-thing into the community that's not already there" (Kukla 1993). Despite this, Commissioners Villani and DeVincenzo voted no on the issue—"The people in the area have suffered enough," the latter explained (Kukla 1993).

In 1995 the Newark City Council sponsored a public forum on the AIDS/HIV virus. Few city officials attended to listen to speakers' concerns. But newly elected councilman Luis Quintana, chair of the HIV/AIDS Planning Committee, was there. He took an active role in the forum, responding to angry residents who asked why no other city health administrators or planning council members had attended. Quintana pledged to investigate why, affirming that their absence was "some kind of disrespect" (Kukla 1995). As Newark's epidemic reached the mid-1990s, he and other local Puerto Rican activists continued to address the impact of HIV/AIDS on the city's Spanish-speaking residents, despite minimal assistance and support.

City officials systematically denied the full extent of Newark's AIDS epidemic, refusing to act when confronted with evidence of the growing threat. Institutional resistance to the wider implications of the epidemic started early. A tense controversy erupted in 1985 when an African American minister proposed that his church fund a homeless shelter for AIDS victims. Rev. David Lee, founder of the House of Refuge Baptist Church, painted a stark picture of PWAs in the city: "Many of these people are out in the street—their families panic and their landlords panic and throw them out. There's just no place for these people to go" (Schulte 1985b). A University Hospital (UMDNJ) doctor, who spoke only on the condition that he remained anonymous, agreed. "On any single day we might have twenty to thirty AIDS or ARC [AIDS-Related Complex, describing late-stage HIV] patients. About a third of them could leave the hospital if they had any place to go." He pointed out that the number of AIDS cases was doubling every six months and it was not likely that the disease would just go away. About the proposed shelter, he said, "Someone has to be thinking in those terms. I don't know who's going to do it—the city, the state, or the county. Someone has to take the responsibility" (Schulte 1985b).

Despite the fact that the proposed shelter was to be located in a square block of abandoned and isolated buildings, Newark city councilman George Branch refused to allow it to be built. "I would oppose a shelter at this time until further discussion with the residents of the ward," he asserted (Schulte 1985b). When questioned, Branch said that he had to consider the interests of the sixty-five hundred people living in the Central Ward as well as the commuters who traveled through it. In the end, he and his supporters succeeded in blocking the shelter, helping to establish the city's response to its HIV-positive citizens for years to come. Advocates and hospital representatives would face absolute resistance from politicians and community leaders as the casualties continued to pile up.

In October of 1986, the state health department tried to open an AIDS unit in a Newark nursing home. When the plan was made public, the outcry was so severe that it was postponed "indefinitely." Shortly after his election, Mayor Sharpe James came out as a key opponent of the proposal. He told reporters that he was "'pleased that the organization . . . ha[d] reconsidered its position' and 'shown their compassion and sensitivity to the community in which they are located' by giving up their bid to establish an AIDS facility" (Whitlow 1986d). Ultimately, the mayor's administration succeeded in blocking the AIDS unit by threatening to rescind a tax abatement previously granted on the building. This caused the developer to back away hurriedly, killing the project.

In July of 1987 the battle began again in earnest. The state announced plans to identify potential long-term care sites, but one of Newark's desperate hospitals could not wait. United Hospital of Newark jumped the gun, attempting to harness the former Park Avenue Hospital for Crippled Children for AIDS care as well as for the care of other chronically ill persons. "I can't wait sixty to ninety days for a study," said UHN president Dr. James R. Cowan. "AIDS is killing my ability to run this hospital" (Whitlow 1987c). Dr. Cowan's sentiments were echoed by Dr. Stanley Bergen of University Hospital (UMDNJ), who explained that his facility was also undergoing increasing financial strain. "We are losing about forty-three hundred to forty-four hundred dollars a day, or about eight thousand to nine thousand dollars for each admission of an AIDS drug abuser" (Narvaez 1987). Newark's hospitals found that they could neither turn PWAs away nor could they afford to treat them.

Despite the hospitals' plea, Newark's director of Health and Welfare refused to support "anything that puts AIDS patients in with senior citizens or anybody else in the same building" (Whitlow 1987c). Callie Foster Shruggs explained that her position was based on the public's perception of AIDS. Shruggs told the press that the city had recently agreed to the creation of two facilities that would serve only AIDS patients—a homeless shelter for those shunned by their families and a nursing home for the terminally ill. The city's administration argued that it was unacceptable to house AIDS patients with HIV-negative patients. Councilwoman Marie Villani articulated this when she commented that "Years ago, tuberculosis patients were isolated in large buildings. . . . People feared tuberculosis then as they do AIDS today. We should look into doing something similar" (Byrd 1988a). The city's administration insisted that all three hospitals share a single chronic care facility for PWAs if they had to create one at all (Whitlow 1987c).

The problem appeared to be one of denial and fear: denial that AIDS was a critical problem in Newark and fear that the city was becoming a dumping ground for AIDS patients (*Star-Ledger* 1987; Byrd 1988a; Boodman 1989). Mayor Sharpe James expressed the latter in his comments about the Park Avenue proposal: "I feel Dr. Molly Coye [health commissioner] and others in Trenton are using Newark as a dumping ground," he charged.

> They are not talking about putting these numbers of beds in other cities. AIDS is a national problem. And to those who say all the AIDS patients are from Newark, I say baloney. They pulled that one on us before, we checked and found it was not true. I condemned the Crippled Children's Hospital proposal when Dr. [James] Cowan brought it to me originally . . . and I condemn this idea. Many hospitals are using the threat of AIDS to get more money. They say they are setting up more space for AIDS patients just to get more money from the state. (*Star-Ledger* 1987)

As mayor, James spearheaded the city's blind institutionalized resistance to the needs of its HIV-positive citizens, but he was not the only one to do so. Councilman Anthony Carrino asserted that the hospital would "open up the AIDS facility at Crippled Children's over my dead body" (Byrd 1988a). State

Senator Ronald L. Rice, also a Newark city councilman, was another official opposed to the AIDS facility. His suspicion that Newark was becoming a repository for AIDS patients led him to introduce legislation requiring that all such patients be treated near their homes. Yet state tracking revealed that the largest number of cases in the state—28 percent—came from Newark and its neighboring municipalities in Essex County (Narvaez 1987).

Not all city officials agreed with Rice and James, but the dumping ground theory acted as a powerful deterrent to change. Dr. Cowan reported that although some officials wanted to support a facility, they feared a public outcry should they approve it, so they took no action (Narvaez 1987). Attempts to open a 125-bed facility in Wanaque later in the year met similar resistance.

Councilman Donald Tucker was one of the few who had supported the Park Avenue proposal completely. Now the chairman of the City Council Committee on AIDS, this former director of addictions services had helped found CURA. Tucker told a *Star-Ledger* reporter that political problems were delaying the creation of an AIDS chronic care center: "I talked with both the Republican and Democratic leadership and they do not wish to be involved on this issue" (Byrd 1988b).

As a result, Newark's PWAs faced homelessness in addition to illness; without long-term care facilities their most basic needs could not be met. Likewise, the city's hospitals found themselves barely able to keep up with the crush of incoming AIDS patients. University Hospital (UMDNJ) responded to the city's wall of resistance through the organization of a conference: "AIDS in Our Community—The Next Victim Could Be You." The plenary speech was given by Dr. Rudolph Jackson, a physician and consultant for the CDC in Atlanta. He had harsh words for his listeners: "For those people who think we don't have a problem, they better get their heads out of the sand . . . the Newark community must be brought together to recognize the gravity of the problem" (Gluck 1987).

As Newark entered 1988, statistics showed that 1,510 new cases of AIDS had been diagnosed during the previous calendar year (Whitlow 1988a). There was no adult treatment or long-term care facility for PWAs in the metropolitan area and no support for additional services within the municipal government. Only a few charitable and service organizations attempted to provide help for families grappling with AIDS. Public perception of Newark's PWAs was at an all-time low and media images of the city's HIV-positive women revolved around drug use, prostitution, and the abuse and abandonment of children.

Despite Newark's harsh and unforgiving climate, Councilman Tucker began speaking to his colleagues about the epidemic. Tucker cited recent research showing that 70 percent of those who had died in Newark had been city residents for at least ten years; he argued against the idea that a Newark AIDS facility would attract nonresidents. "The overwhelming majority of those dying from this disease are Newarkers," he insisted (Byrd 1988c). Tucker produced the data to back up his argument, especially a report prepared for the Department of Health that laid out the sizable costs of Newark's minimalist and haphazard approach to AIDS care.

Perhaps swayed by his compelling economic analysis, Mayor Sharpe James finally agreed to meet with five hospital CEOs from Newark hospitals shortly thereafter in order to explore the possibility of establishing an adult AIDS-care facility (Byrd 1988c). After the meeting, James changed his position completely. He announced that he was *in favor* of establishing a long-term care facility "for persons suffering from AIDS . . . we cannot bury our heads in the sand on this issue . . . I will meet with the city council and we must take a leadership position in addressing this most pressing need" (Byrd 1988d).

At the same time, Tucker helped organize a community forum on the AIDS crisis (Byrd 1988e; Byrd 1988f). Two recommendations resulted from the gathering: that one hundred thousand dollars of the city budget be used to hire two AIDS counselors and support staff, and that a site be found for a sub-acute facility to care for AIDS patients who were not yet in need of hospitalization. At the forum, Tucker pressed his agenda further, publicizing the work of a new, informal AIDS speaker's bureau of at least thirty-five individuals. "We want to send speakers to all community groups in the city to spread information about the disease and combat the hysteria we've been seeing," he said. The bureau had already begun organizing informational workshops in Newark area churches, community centers, and block association meetings. Tucker greatly encouraged forum participants to become involved in this grassroots educational effort. He described a new, fledgling interest among city residents in the local AIDS epidemic: "This is a break in the attitude we saw before of people saying they would not discuss or interact with the disease. People are ready now," he said (Byrd 1988f).

By early spring of 1989, multiple voices sought to represent the concerns of Newark's PWAs. Derek Winans, founder of the year-old Newark Community Project for People with AIDS, spoke at a congressional hearing held at Essex County College in an attempt to generate funds for the city's AIDS-related efforts (Boodman 1989). The hearing, "AIDS—Planning for the Next 10 Years," had been organized by Representative Donald Payne to outline the greatest areas of need and generate new strategies for meeting them. At the hearing, Winans explained that Newark's response to the epidemic lagged behind other urban centers by about five years at best, and that the community had long been entrenched in a state of denial about the epidemic (Phipps 1989).

Union Hospital's AIDS coordinator, Edward Szmitkowski, also testified that the city needed an AIDS resource directory and both interim and permanent housing for the infected. "If you don't have good nutrition or hygiene or a place to lay your head at night, you can't avoid being sick. In New York, there's a place called Bailey House on Christopher Street where ambulatory patients can go if they've been evicted. There's no place like that here in Newark" (Phipps 1989).

By the end of the month, Governor Jim Florio approved an emergency rule accelerating the rate at which the State Department of Health could review and grant requests to build community-based homes and long-term care facilities for people with AIDS. Now, applications were to be reviewed on a monthly basis. This decision addressed the fact that only 120 long-term care beds in the state were set aside to serve an estimated forty thousand HIV-positive New Jersey residents, ten thousand of whom had been diagnosed with AIDS. Florio also emphasized the importance of addressing the unmet need for AIDS-related non-hospital services (*Star-Ledger* 1990).

Just when it appeared that state and municipal denial of the AIDS epidemic was changing, Joan Whitlow, a *Star-Ledger* reporter who covered HIV/AIDS, helped break some bad news:

> Some $5 million in federal AIDS money for northern New Jersey has been lost because the city of Newark, the pipeline for the grants, failed to distribute on time $2.6 million already allocated for the region, officials announced yesterday. In addition to Newark, the money would have helped East Orange, Irvington, and Morris, Sussex, Warren, and Union counties. Those areas are in a pool funded by the Ryan White Title I Care and Treatment Act grant for the region, which has Newark Mayor Sharpe James listed as the principal grantee. . . . The Newark City Council, which must approve the Ryan White contracts for the region, approved the first twenty-eight for 1992 only two weeks ago and there are seventeen more contracts to go to fully allocate the 1993 funds . . . the city does not have the money in hand. . . . [Bobi] Ruffin [Newark's Department of Health and Human Services director] said the local agencies from major hospitals to community groups, have been managing to provide services on their own and would receive money retroactively from the city. Asked how the agencies managed, she said, "I cannot answer that question." (Whitlow 1993)

Denise Cole, a volunteer social worker for the New Jersey Chapter of Today's Woman, revealed that HIV Planning Council members had allowed Bobi Ruffin, Newark's Department of Health and Human Services director, to take funds from impoverished urban social service organizations and reallocate them to a few large hospitals and institutions serving suburban and upper-income families. The planning council power struggle had kept many of Newark's small CBOs from accessing the funds they needed to meet the needs of local AIDS-affected families (Wilson 1992). The scandal was tremendous.

Criticisms of the mayor, the council, and the co-chairs flew back and forth with lightening speed: "It is our sons, our daughters, our friends who are going to die" without the needed services, said Union County HIV Consortium chair Mary E. Kelly (Whitlow 1993).

Mayor Sharpe James was furious and resolved to replace half the council immediately, but the acting council chairman threatened to go to court to stop him if he did so (Whitlow 1993). By the second week of April, Newark had applied for discretionary funds to avoid interruption of services, and the swearing in of replacement council members had begun (Walker 1993a; Walker 1993b). By May, nine original members had been replaced, but the city was embroiled in an all-out court battle over the dismissal of two other former council members (Walker 1993c). In June, a federal judge upheld the mayor's right to replace the council but strongly condemned all parties for their inaction and their failure to provide assistance to people with AIDS. Most tellingly, the judge said that area AIDS patients had been seriously hampered in their efforts to access benefits by "monstrous administrative tangles"; he placed the "primary responsibility" for this at the mayor's door (Rudolph 1993).

Confronted by the staggering costs of their refusal to act, the city's administration had no choice but to begin the slow process of change. Newark's 1995 resubmission for federal funding was partially successful—the region received $6.2 million with which to serve its growing number of HIV-positive residents— sixty-six hundred of which had been diagnosed with AIDS (Whitlow 1995b). When most of the women in my study began searching for help in the mid-1990s, the city had just begun to turn itself around.

The AIDS epidemic unfolded differently in Newark than it did in other parts of the country because city residents had little access to cultural and social capital capable of overcoming institutionalized resistance. In 1986, Margaret Nichols, executive director of the Hyacinth Foundation, explained why so many of New Jersey's PWAs found themselves locked out of Manhattan's clinical drug trials. As the head of a service organization that served people with AIDS, she had a great deal of exposure to the problem. In her view, the problem lay with the limited social networks of local PWAs. "New Jerseyans often have a difficult time getting into programs in other states," she said. "It's a matter of being in the right place at the right time, of knowing someone who knows that there are eight places open [in a clinical trial] and they will be filled by eight o'clock. Just knowing another person with AIDS in such a program helps. . . . And you hear of people who work in the New York hospitals which are doing research getting their friends in. The process is one of who you know gets you in, and let's face it, that benefits white, middle-class [gay] men" (Whitlow 1986b).

Newark's PWAs were not gay white men with political connections—they were African Americans and Puerto Ricans living in the state's poorest urban center. As impoverished IV drug users and their partners, they often depended on hospital emergency rooms for their care. Without the ability to forge relationships with gatekeepers of cutting-edge medicine, they had no choice but to depend on whatever the city could scrape together. "As a group, drug users lack the social and legal organizations which have formed around gay rights issues," Nichols explained. "And the social and economic status of drug users is usually such that they are not easily able to move through a health research system where *who you know becomes a matter of survival*" (Whitlow 1986b).

The experiences of New Jersey residents who got into clinical trials supported this analysis. Robert Negran, a New Brunswick man participating in Sloan-Kettering's trials, confirmed that it was partly a matter of knowing the right people. In his case, his partner, a doctor, arranged a New York consultation immediately after his diagnosis. Negran was referred to Sloan-Kettering, and his admission into the first trial positioned him to get into others. As a well-connected PWA, he commented, "You know what is going on. You develop a rapport with doctors, and when a new program comes up, it is easier to find out about it" (Whitlow 1986c). But without the opportunity to create rapport with the professionals running the trials, Newark's PWAs were excluded from the process.

At every level, Newark's marginalized PWAs found themselves shut off from cutting-edge AIDS treatment. Even the presumably unbiased National Institutes of Health (NIH) overlooked New Jersey in its original distribution of AIDS grant money, much to the shock of clinical practitioners drowning in Newark's epidemic. Pediatric specialist James Oleske was appalled when his coalition of hospitals failed to land a national grant that would have helped house, treat, and counsel Newark's AIDS patients. "When they gave out fourteen [grants]—and to places like Rochester, NY, which has no AIDS patients to speak of, I'm in a state of shock," he told a local journalist (Whitlow 1986b).

In August of 1988, a group of forty New Jersey AIDS advocacy groups formed the North Jersey Community Research Initiative (NJCRI), an unorthodox research institute. Their network of community-based clinics and physicians began conducting their own research studies. Bill Orr, the executive director of NJCRI, came from New Jersey's ACT UP coalition. He brought the resources, expertise, and social networks of New York's sophisticated AIDS community into Newark's struggle. Orr drew on allies like Jeff Bomser, another NJCRI board member, who could share his expertise in complementary and alternative medicine (CAM) with the Newark community.

In a *Star-Ledger* newspaper article, Bomser outlined an important CAM treatment strategy commonly used by upper- and middle-class PWAs: the use of HIV/AIDS-focused, member-run buyers' clubs (Whitlow 1988b). These clubs negotiated directly with U.S. and European drug and herb suppliers in order to gain access to experimental treatment substances at highly reduced prices. This created a "gray market" through which club members could design "integrative" (referring to a combination of biomedical and CAM) treatment plans and help direct their own care ("integrative medicine" refers to the combination of conventional and alternative modalities in an effort to address the biological, psychological, social, and spiritual aspects of health and illness) (Rees 2001).

In the interview, Bomser described some of the complementary and alternative treatments that he acquired through buyers' clubs. For example, he bought soy lecithin and mixed it with melted butter and water in his kitchen to produce homemade AL-721, an expensive experimental treatment. He also acknowledged that those who couldn't afford this kind of therapy—like Newark's poor PWAs—simply did not get it. "I can't tell a PWA from Newark or New Jersey that we are fighting the same battle because we are not. And we should be" (Whitlow 1988b).

Bomser and Orr emphasized the need to expand treatment options for all of Newark's PWAs. For example, Orr explained that most research programs typically did not admit women because of the fear that they would become pregnant and expose their fetus to experimental drugs. But in Newark and New Jersey, women made up one of the fastest-growing segments of the population living with HIV/AIDS. NJCRI decided to include them in every study (Whitlow 1988b). The institute would attack New Jersey's vast HIV/AIDS treatment inequities and provide the first real remedy to Newark's lack of access to private doctors, clinical trials, experimental treatments, and CAM strategies.

In 1995, Newark officials asked for $8.3 million in federal grants. This fell far short of the $18 million actually needed, according to the most recent needs assessment survey (Whitlow 1995a). Charles Jones, director of the Union County HIV Consortium, pointed out that Newark's Eligible Metropolitan Area (NEMA) had suffered because it lacked the well-organized AIDS groups so common in other high-caseload EMAs. Like others working with the Newark's AIDS community, Jones explained that cities like San Francisco, Los Angeles, and New York had benefited from the organizational efforts—and higher economic status—of gay activists there (Boodman 1989; Hancock 2002). "If the things that happened to this EMA in the last few years had happened in New York, the AIDS community there would have been out in force. . . . New York City received more money than they requested last year. I'm not saying that they can't make use of it, but this EMA could have used more money" (Whitlow 1995a). But because Newark's residents lacked the middle-class cultural and social capital that translated into economic leverage, the city's AIDS coalitions were at a tremendous disadvantage as they tried to compete for resources and funding.

As Caridad and her peers began looking for help, the city had just begun to offer services for women living with the virus. Decades of political foot-dragging and selective blindness had hampered the development of a broad, well-funded resource base for people living with HIV/AIDS. Women like Nini, Deborah, and Julia could draw on broad cultural capital to help build the relationships—or social capital—required to extract the resources they needed. But for women like Amelia, Nilsa, and Carlotta, who depended only on their native cultural capital, the task was much harder.

4

Understanding HIV

The women I worked with all had acquaintances, friends, and even family members who had contracted the virus, but they were unprepared to hear the diagnosis themselves. HIV/AIDS was something that happened to other people. They had all been exposed to both the national and local discourse about AIDS—group discussions, statements, and opinions about it, media broadcasts on HIV (like talk show segments or TV newscasts), and newspapers and magazine articles. But once each woman began struggling with the illness herself, she started to draw on what she had heard and what she believed in order to make sense of what was happening. In essence, each woman had to develop a new relationship with HIV to incorporate it into her own worldview.

Understanding what HIV came to mean to women engaged in this process was an important part of understanding their survival strategies. I used a series of questions known as Explanatory Model questions to explore these meanings. They were originally developed by psychiatrist and medical anthropologist Arthur Kleinman to help health care professionals understand their patients' illness and health beliefs. Taken together, the questions can help clarify how people understand and relate to their illnesses (Kleinman 1988).

Kleinman describes *explanatory models* as

> notions that patients, families, and practitioners have about a specific illness episode. These informal descriptions of what an illness is about have enormous clinical significance: to ignore them may be fatal. They respond to such questions as, What is the nature of this problem? Why has it affected me? Why now? What course will it follow? How does it most affect my body? What treatments do I desire? What do I most fear about the illness and its treatment? Explanatory models are responses to urgent

life circumstances . . . [that] contain contradictions and shift in content. They are our representations of the cultural flow of life experience: consequently . . . they congeal and unravel as that flow and our understanding of it firms up in one situation only to dissolve in another. (Kleinman 1988, 120–122)

I asked the Explanatory Model questions at the close of each woman's first semistructured interview. After all interviews were transcribed, I coded them in a qualitative software program called NUDIST, grouping responses to each question together and noting emerging themes. As I explored the patterns that emerged, I attempted to preserve women's voices whenever possible, illustrating each theme with their own words.

Variations of the questions have emerged. The precise form in which they are asked is flexible (Fadiman 1997). As long as core issues are addressed in sequence, the format is fluid. In my interviews, I chose to use a simplified version (Kleinman 1980). The first, "What do you call your problem?" encouraged women to tell me about both medical and slang terms for HIV and AIDS. Their answers gave me a sense of how they saw the virus and what kind of relationship they expected to have with it. When I asked, "What do you think caused the problem?" most women answered as if I had asked, "Did sex or drugs infect you? Exactly how did it happen?" A few women, however, offered me their theories about how the virus itself originated, telling me both their personal stories and their interpretations of how it entered their communities.

Because symptoms of HIV infection can manifest years after the actual moment of infection, the question "Why do you think your symptoms started when they did?" provoked thoughtful reflection about their first moments of awareness that something was wrong with their bodies. For some women, the question provoked heated discussions of medication side effects; for others, it led to the sharing of theories about why they began experiencing symptoms when they did or why they were still asymptomatic.

I asked the next set of questions in order to explore each woman's daily experience of HIV, her views about the illness itself, and her expectations for her future: "What do you think the illness does to you? How does it work? How severe is it? Will it have a long or short course? What do you fear most about it? What are the chief problems it causes in your life?" Their answers revealed some of the most basic ways in which HIV shaped their lives. Most poignantly, it emphasized the ways in which their physical symptoms proved less troubling than the effects of HIV-related stigma.

"What kind of treatments do you think you should receive? What results do you want the most?" targeted their attitudes toward the treatment options available to them and elicited their opinions of the regimens they had been prescribed. And although most wanted a cure more than anything else, not every woman did. This was a surprise, as was the critically important role of treatment in suppressing all outward signs of illness.

What Do You Call Your Problem?

Eight women used the terms "HIV," "HIV-positive," or "SIDA" (the Spanish acronym for AIDS) most of the time when discussing their illness. Two also spoke about "the virus." The latter was the term I heard used most often in support groups and social service agencies. All of these labels invoke medical models; they are used in the media and in scientific and popular publications of all kinds. Because they are part of the standardized discourse around HIV/AIDS, it was no surprise that women used them so frequently. Yet they were not the only ones in use.

The Monster

Caridad, Nilsa, and Amelia each mentioned that HIV was often called "el monstruo," or "the monster" in their neighborhoods and social circles. Sometimes it was "el monstruo verde," "the green monster." Nilsa told me that it was common to hear people talk about the virus in this way. "We often use the expression 'the monster,'" she explained. "You hear a lot of people saying, 'Oh, el monstruo is killing me—this monster is killing me.'" Here, HIV is depicted as a predator destroying those who stumble into its path. This metaphor imagines HIV-positive women to be helpless victims who can't free themselves from its deadly grasp. Although they might fend off an attack here and there, the term suggests that its victims are forever in danger of surrendering to a power greater than themselves, and eventually, they will fall before it.

Perhaps because of these implicit meanings, not everyone approved of the term. When I asked Nini what she called the problem, she made a point of saying, "I *don't* call it 'the monster' like others do; I try to avoid that." This was well in keeping with her resistance to most aspects of the sick role. The term "sick role" refers to a temporary identity adopted by or imposed on those who are ill. Generally, it exempts the ill person from their usual social roles and responsibilities and stresses the need for rest and recuperation (Larson 2009). Nini insisted that she, not some disease, controlled her destiny. Yet even she was not immune to the perception that HIV was a killer stalking her from behind. Very occasionally, she referred to the virus as "my death sentence." And although "el monstruo" was the most common metaphor used to describe HIV, it was not the only one. Amelia had her own name for the monster—she told me that she sometimes called it "Pac Man," because "it does eat you from the inside, and it's always eating you little by little, as I call it."

Emphasizing the Sick Role

Not everyone focused on the monstrous nature of the virus. Many women preferred to emphasize that HIV was simply an illness when they talked about it themselves. When I asked Flor to name her problem, she shrugged her shoulders and explained that she said "I am infected" ("yo estoy infectada") whenever the subject came up. If others didn't understand what she meant by that, she would follow it up by saying, "I'm positive HIV [*sic*]." In a similar vein, Gabrielle preferred to say that that she was "enfermita," a Spanish term meaning "ill" that softened the nature of the illness through the use of the diminutive suffix "ita." Adding "ita" to a subject suggests that it is smaller, less threatening ,or even more endearing than it would otherwise be. She translated "enfermita" literally as "sicky," a word that puzzled her English-speaking friends. Both women used terms that emphasized physical frailty, suggesting adoption of the sick role. Neither approach suggested that HIV was anything other than an illness: another physical condition that sometimes limited or affected what they could do. Each term was remarkably neutral, unlike the term "monster."

Carlotta took a third approach. She avoided calling the virus anything at all. In fact, she said she never spoke about it to anyone. Amelia and Gabrielle echoed this sentiment. Initially, Amelia said she avoided referring to HIV at all or just called it "this thing," and Gabrielle told me that she never talked about it. Amelia and Gabrielle eventually articulated at least one label that they sometimes used. Carlotta never did. After several discussions, I realized that I had rarely, if ever, heard her refer to the virus by name. In the course of our conversations, she told me that the most specific thing she would ever say to a friend or family member about HIV would be, "Well, with today's bad situation, one must use condoms." I also noted this unwillingness to name the condition in Paquita, who spent many days with me over a stretch of several months without once naming her illness.

Not surprisingly, Carlotta and Paquita were highly secretive about their condition: they were among the most closeted women in my study. Neither woman considered herself a member of Newark's AIDS community and neither participated in HIV-related workshops, social activities, or educational efforts. However, their caution was nowhere so evident as in the words they did not say and the names they would not speak.

Although Carlotta was unwilling to call her illness by any name, she was willing to talk about her perceptions. She explained her thoughts of HIV/AIDS as "un descuidado," the result of an act of carelessness or neglect. Her willingness to discuss the impact of HIV on her life and private thoughts made clear her frequent self-reflection, even though she kept quiet most of the time. The contrast between her public silence and her private musings was striking, as was the way in which she bounded her discussions of HIV, only once mentioning the role of anyone else in its transmission.

I wondered if Carlotta felt responsible for contracting HIV. She emphasized the fact that she contracted the virus through sex, but spoke only in reference to herself. For her, HIV seemed to be the outcome of a decision she herself had made—and one that she regretted.

Like Carlotta, Nerina distinguished between speaking publicly and reflecting privately: "In my mind, I call it 'AIDS,' but I *say* 'the virus.'" Perhaps AIDS, with its terrifying connotations, was too dreadful to say in public. But Nerina did not try to hide her status. She was not in the closet. As a frequent participant in HIV-related support groups and workshops, she was a mainstay of her local AIDS community. Like her peers, she adopted the relatively neutral term "virus" for everyday conversation rather than using the stigmatizing term "AIDS." Yet, as a person who had been living with AIDS since her first HIV test, she knew what she had, and it wasn't just "the virus"; it was an advanced form of the disease. Nerina took more responsibility for self-care than anyone else I met in the AIDS community. She monitored her diet meticulously, took a huge array of supplements, and was always on the lookout for another set of behavioral changes that could prolong the length and quality of her life. For her, an AIDS diagnosis reinforced self-care rather than promoting despair. "It makes me stronger . . . prayer, massages, moving . . . I boost the [power of the] prayers by vitamins and juicing . . . it makes me stronger."

An Alternative Model of Illness

As one of two active members of NA (Narcotics Anonymous) in my study, Deborah adopted a different approach. NA, an outgrowth of AA (Alcoholics Anonymous), is an international organization of affiliated community groups that help former narcotics users recover from addiction and maintain sobriety. Deborah used the NA framework and its terminology to help her interpret HIV. When I asked what she called her problem, she said that she often spoke about "HIV" or "the virus," but sometimes called it "the second disease":

> In NA they call it the first disease and the second disease . . . when we're sharing and stuff like that, we tell them that sometimes we have partners but like we're living with both diseases and when we pray, we pray for the still sick and suffering and those who are living in and outside the room, living by the *first disease*, which is either relapse or recovery, or the *second disease*, which is AIDS and HIV.

In this model, HIV is secondary to addiction, the central problem of NA group members. Addiction is the illness they attempt to keep under control. "Recovery" is a term used by NA and related groups like AA to mean the process of learning to free one's self from active addiction. HIV is a secondary challenge. This made sense to Deborah. She believed that while it was important to monitor her health and control the level of virus in her bloodstream, her first priority was to stay in recovery. "The first, most important thing is not to pick up . . . I'm going to go talk to a group [today] . . . and telling them how I crossed that wall to give them hope. I'm gonna try to help them, to show them the tools to use so you don't pick up. It's when you stop using your tools that you fall." Deborah assembled a broad range of social support strategies to help her meet this goal. She attended NA meetings, spoke frequently with her sponsor, leaned on non-NA friends, and worked with two mental health professionals. She used this support network to make sure that she never got so overwhelmed that she returned to drugs. For Deborah, HIV was serious, but relapsing into addiction was what she feared the most.

What Do You Think Caused Your Problem?

Personal Explanations

Nine women answered this question by telling me that their husbands or long-term partners had infected them. Nini told me that she contracted the virus from "my ex-husband—I *know* he got it and gave it to me. I *know*, and that makes it worse." Or as Alicia put it, "[I got it] from unprotected sex with my husband. He brought it home. I didn't have to go and get it." This aware-ness was accompanied by anger: "I was not looking for this. I was legally married. I was not at risk. No drinking or drugs, no going out, no playing around." Some husbands, like Nini's, *knew* they were HIV-positive before the start of the relation-ship but did not reveal this. In others, partners probably contracted the virus during the course of the relationship, but kept it a secret. In Celestina's case, Roberto *did* disclose his status immediately upon learning it, but by then it was too late.

Women like Nini, Amelia, and Nilsa, who believed they were consciously deceived, expressed the most anger. They shook with rage when they talked about their husbands. Others spoke with resignation. Juana and Deborah thought they might have contracted the virus from either a boyfriend or from trading sex for money during hard times; both expressed more regret than anger. All, however, struggled to manage the emotions provoked by their experiences.

Structural Explanations

Not everyone thought about their risks in such an individual, personalized way. Gabrielle, for example, offered a holistic perspective about her encounter with the virus.

GABRIELLE: My lifestyle brought me to this place. It brought me to drug abuse. It brought me to AIDS. My style of life cost me my children. I am screwed because of my lifestyle.

SABRINA: But you are talking about it in the big picture.

GABRIELLE: As a whole, as a whole, very simple . . . because I am not going to think that if I was a different person I wouldn't have got it, cause I never thought about being somebody else.

She insisted that the structure of her life as a whole had brought the virus to her door. This vision is similar to that of theorists like Merrill Singer, who argue that the SAVA syndemic, which intertwines substance abuse, violence, and HIV/AIDS so tightly, is the true cause of our urban HIV epidemic. He argues that it is a mistake to examine each of these factors in isolation. Paul Farmer tells us that these larger factors are what put women, in particular, at risk (Farmer, Simmons, and Connors 1996). Gabrielle denied she could disaggregate her experience, her "risks," down to a few key moments or isolated decisions. Doing so misrepresented the truth of her life.

Selma and Julia also offered more global perspectives about the source of their illness. Instead of focusing on how they *personally* contracted HIV, they suspected that the virus itself was a human creation, born from a government plan or experiment.

I kind of doubt a lot of times, you know, versions and histories that I hear? When people say that it was created by the government or something, . . . I don't go for it all the way, but because of the government have had a lot of laxing in investigation and researching that pushes me to feel that there is a conspiracy or something.

Here, Julia is considering the possibility that she and her community are victims of a government conspiracy. Instead of laying the underlying responsibility on a partner, drugs, or structural issues, she is willing to at least entertain the notion that she is just one more victim of a government plot. While she does not say that the motivation for this crime is the government's desire to rid itself of undesirables, this is implicit in her argument. Ineffective and irresolute government responses to HIV/AIDS only strengthen her suspicions.

Julia stops just short of saying that HIV is a tool of the elite, intended for the underclass. Selma does not: "White men put something together and gave it to a group of people, and . . . this is what I believe . . . gave it to a group of people and didn't care, did not care what anybody else was gonna feel or how they were gonna feel. It is a man-made, actually a man-made disease." Although Selma blames a former partner for her immediate illness, as noted in her biographical sketch, she suspects the underlying cause may be a Tuskegee-like experiment through which the virus was introduced into her community. From 1932 to 1972, the U.S. Public Health Service conducted the Tuskegee syphilis study on a group of poor African American farmers. The men were never told about their illness and were prevented from receiving curative treatment when it became available (Jones 1981). I encountered this belief from time to time in waiting-room conversations and gatherings that took place in Newark's AIDS community. Michele Berger also encountered conspiracy theories around HIV in her study of HIV-positive African American women living in Detroit (Berger 2004).

Why Did Your Symptoms Start When They Did?

Physiological Explanations

Answers to this question varied, depending on women's experience of HIV-related symptoms and medication side effects. Alicia, Amelia, Juana, and Luchita all told me that they had problems only after taking HIV medications and rarely experienced HIV-related symptoms. Alicia spoke for several when she said, "[The medications] make me tired, constantly tired, my body aches. You know, I don't have the energies to get up and go. But other people, forget it, they are getting all the side effects." All but Juana made a point of telling me that medication side effects were very debilitating. Nerina, Celestina, Nilsa, and Nini, who lived with many HIV-related symptoms, explained that medication side effects made it impossible to adhere to their medication regimen perfectly. Nerina and Celestina experienced side effects so traumatic that they were unwilling to take HIV medications at all despite signs of disease progression. Nerina explained, "I've been undetectable. [Nerina's "undetectable" refers to the point at which levels of HIV RNA in the blood are too low to be detected with a viral load test (AIDS Info Glossary).]And without protease inhibitors. Just by my diet, my herbs and things, my cleansing out, and everything. I've been undetectable twice, and the medications have messed me up bad . . . they try and kill me with this stuff, you know what I'm saying?" The experience of side effects was almost universal, although Caridad and Flor experienced no side effects or symptoms at all. But for most, medication side effects were an important marker of HIV and it was extremely common for the women to point to medications, rather than the disease itself, as the central source of their physical distress.

Psychological Explanations

Two women saw another reason for the emergence of their symptoms: the fear and the psychological trauma they experienced at diagnosis. Deborah links the two in her story about the moment she learned the truth.

SABRINA: When did you start having symptoms?

DEBORAH: [laughing] As soon as they told me. I thought I was dying. I thought I was gonna die.

SABRINA: Why do you think that happened?

DEBORAH: Because I wasn't educated on it. They just came out and they just told me and then they got a social worker and she explained to me what it was and she told me to take these pills, that I was gonna be OK, that it's, like, I was a carrier, and I was living with it, and that I was gonna be fine. And that was that. But my first instinct was, I banged my head against the wall and I was, like, "I'm gonna die. I'm gonna die."

SABRINA: So why do you think you got the first symptoms when you did?

DEBORAH: My mind

SABRINA: Your mind?

DEBORAH: I actually assumed that I was gonna die because I wasn't educated on it.

Deborah believed that the fear of death provoked her symptoms. After learning more about the virus, and especially after meeting healthy HIV-positive individuals, her symptoms resolved. More than anything else, she said, she needed role models who were successfully managing the disease and could teach her to do the same. Because she sought out support groups and social service agencies, she was able to meet an entire community of people who were managing HIV successfully. Always the grassroots activist, Deborah translated her personal experience into social commentary; she was eager to share her ideas about how to prevent what happened to her from happening to anyone else.

I *strongly* believe that they should have TV commercials on TV educating people about the virus and not discriminate it as a sickness or terminally ill thing. They should put it, like, you can live with it, you know. Like you know how they have these breast cancer commercials and ads and stuff like this . . . and I also strongly believe that if they were to have commercials showing a pregnant mother, OK, holding her belly, holding her unborn child, and letting herself know that she's gonna be OK and her baby is gonna be OK, that everything is gonna be OK, you know.

Between public service announcements, daytime dramas, and talk shows, Deborah suggested, women could be taught that HIV was a manageable chronic disease rather than a death sentence. I saw many of the women in my study watching daytime dramas, so I suspect she was right. Like early gay activists, Deborah said that mislabeling HIV was as costly as the virus itself. She also laid the responsibility for accurate public health campaigns at the feet of government officials, just as gay activists had once done.

Nilsa also thought her symptoms might have a psychological root. She told me, "I don't know why [they started when they did]—maybe it's in my mind, because the mind starts creating things when you begin to imagine a bit about what is happening." Nilsa felt ambivalent about this possibility, however.

She deeply resented the doctors who had suggested that her migraines might be psychosomatic. The headaches arrived unpredictably and left her nearly paralyzed. She linked them to a bump that had appeared at the base of her scalp after her diagnosis. Nilsa had shown the lump to her doctors, but they expressed no connection between it and her pain. Although she sometimes insisted that both the bump and her headaches were linked to HIV, at other times she vacillated, wondering if they were symptoms of emotional anguish.

Spiritual Explanations

Both Julia and Gabrielle offered me spiritual explanations for the appearance of their symptoms. Julia explained that "at that time, spiritually, I believe it was like a wake-up call, you know, because I was [taking] certain, like taking medications and stuff like that." Gabrielle attributed the emergence of her symptoms to a force greater than herself: "It was time. I was getting them. It was time . . . it was time for my body to break down." Both thought their symptoms were manifestations of some higher power—either God or destiny, and that something greater than disease acceleration was at work.

Neither woman saw her symptoms as overly negative. In one case, they were almost a blessing, and in the other, they were interpreted as neutral fact. Even though Gabrielle thought that her body was breaking down, she also believed that HIV had been a good influence on her life, an interpretation we will explore later. Because of this, her symptoms, while unpleasant, were not horrifying to her.

What Does It Do to You? How Does It Work?

Physical Symptoms

Six women told me that their energy levels had dropped dramatically as a result of their illness. This was by far the most widely reported problem. Even those denying other symptoms said that the virus had lowered their energy levels. Cristina, Caridad, and Juana all belonged to this low-energy yet asymptomatic group. When I asked whether or not they were affected by the virus, some thought fatigue might be a result of HIV medications (a problem noted previously) rather than the virus itself.

Five women reported clear symptoms. Alicia and Carlotta discovered their seropositive status following experience of symptoms. Alicia's face and eyes swelled up to huge proportions and Carlotta began getting rashes all over her legs. For Alicia, the immediate culprit was toxoplasmosis. Her diagnosis tipped off an emergency room physician, and the results came back positive. Carlotta noticed red spots that looked like mosquito bites on her legs. She also struggled with lypodystrophy—her arms became thin, while her belly expanded and refused to get smaller no matter what she did. Nilsa battled frequent migraine headaches and Deborah acquired a serious thrush infection in her throat. Finally, Nerina experienced a whole host of symptoms: persistent neuropathy that meant she now had to use a cane; forgetfulness and confusion; and nose bleeds and periodic pneumocystic carinii pneumonia (PCP) infections. (PCP is a life-threatening form of pneumonia common among people with suppressed immune systems or autoimmune disorders [AIDS Info Glossary].)

Depression: An Unmentioned Problem

Only two women mentioned depression when answering this question. This was a surprise, since ten had referred to it in other conversations. Nine of these women had sought help to deal with the problem. Most tried support groups, agency-sponsored therapy, or consultations with ministers and priests. For some women, these options were useful, but not everyone was satisfied, as in Paquita's case. As noted previously, Paquita was never able to access mental health services with which she felt comfortable, and her depression remained untreated.

Radical Life Change

Nilsa, Nini, and Gabrielle responded by explaining that HIV had radically changed their lives. Nilsa and Nini saw this as a curse and Gabrielle as a blessing. Both of the former struggled with depression after their diagnoses; the latter did not. All three experienced HIV-related symptoms as well as medication side effects, but HIV's most profound impact was in the way it reshaped their choices. Nilsa explained, "[The diagnosis of HIV] changes your whole life. You're not the same woman. It affects a person's mind the most, you know." Similarly, Nini said,

> It changed my life—I don't see things like I used to. I used to have dreams. By now I would have had a house, I was gonna have a car, my kid was gonna go to a good high school—life would have been like a normal human being. [But now] no matter how much I try, it's impossible. But my life is more normal than others [who have the virus].

Their physical suffering was hard, but the loss of hope imposed an even greater burden. Both women experienced periods of depression, but they handled it in different ways: Nilsa stayed close to home, limiting her activities and interactions, while Nini aggressively pursued all available treatments and resources. Yet each woman articulated the same anguish as she reflected on her lost future.

But Gabrielle saw her new life as a gift: "It made me a better person . . . this sickness has helped me to be a better person and to change." Unlike Nilsa and Nini, Gabrielle had never foreseen a future with a stable life, a family, and a steady partner. Because she spent so much time in jail and on the street, her expectations had been low. HIV forced her to stop and rethink her choices, which resulted in a complete reorientation of her life. In order to live longer, she decided to get an apartment. She began staying off the streets, getting regular rest, and spending time with her granddaughter. She started eating fresh vegetables and wholesome foods and making regular clinic visits. Finally, she began working hand-in-hand with a doctor she trusted to create a treatment plan she could live with. HIV inspired Gabrielle to re-create her life in a more satisfying way. Instead of stealing away her bright future, it gave her a new lease on life.

How Severe Is It? Will It Have a Long or Short Course?

Guarded Optimism

Almost every woman I spoke to agreed that HIV was very serious. Amelia poignantly described the way she moved from the belief that HIV was a death sentence to the realization that it could be a manageable chronic condition. "At the beginning, it was very serious to me. I seen myself in a coffin, I seen my kids without a mother—but now, there's so many medicines, it's like any other disease—people know about it, it's not like they look at you like a monster. [It's] more like cancer."

Despite her initial fear and depression, Amelia came to believe that HIV was a manageable part of her life. Most of the women I worked with agreed with her, but were divided on what that meant for them. Several thought that they were in a better position to stay healthy and live longer than other HIV-positive people. Interestingly, neither symptom severity nor disease stage predicted whether or not a woman would be this optimistic. Caridad, who was completely asymptomatic and had been told that she had a nonprogressive form of the virus, explained that: "Yes, it's serious. Very serious. But for me, for me it's not serious. I am already used to it. I am going to be here for many years, I'm going to see my grandchildren and everything."

Given her lack of symptoms and excellent prognosis, this belief was understandable. But Nerina, who had been diagnosed with AIDS from the start, also took an optimistic stance. "I'm [diagnosed as having] AIDS. So . . . not as serious as them guys, some people have zero T-cells. At least I have, 250 . . . Dr. Fitzgerald said I went as low as 1 . . . and, uh, I've been undetectable. . . . I'm gonna be around for a long while." T-cells are a type of disease-fighting white blood cell critical to the body's immune system (AIDS Info Glossary). As it happened, she lived only three more years, and during those years, she was hospitalized on multiple occasions.

Carlotta also believed that she was protected from the worst HIV could offer, despite daily struggles against stigmatization, lypodystrophy, swollen legs, and skin rashes:

It's very serious. When you contract this illness everyone cuts you off. Another reason is that it deforms your body. If you don't take care of

yourself, it will quickly, quickly finish you off. But if you take care of
yourself and behave well, if you take your medicines calmly, you can last
a little longer than . . . [chuckles]

Here, Carlotta voices a common opinion: while HIV and AIDS were serious,
some women believed they could live long lives if they found ways to cope with
their challenges. Alicia offered me a pragmatic analysis of her condition and the
attitude it demanded of her on a day-to-day basis.

It's something real, real serious, but you know my attitude is, I have it,
I know, but you know I have to deal with it. Like, something I have to do
every day . . . so, how I take it? You don't see me depressed because of
this . . . sitting down thinking I'm gonna die, NO! Uh uh.

Deborah took a similar approach, insisting that what mattered was the way
she met the challenge: "It's bad—some people can deal with it, some can't. *I* ain't
going nowhere." Both women felt that their attitudes and health management
practices were the most important influences on their health. Interestingly,
both followed their drug regimens as well as exploring CAM (complementary
and alternative medicine) treatment options.

Only one person, Selma, said that HIV was "not serious," and she was
careful to qualify her position. For her, viral load was what distinguished a
serious case of HIV from a moderate one: "It's not serious at all. It's serious
where I have to protect myself, to protect others, to protect my family, but it's
not serious where—I wasn't diagnosed [as having AIDS] and they always take my
blood test; it's not there. So they can't detect it."

Selma believed that her illness was not serious as long as her viral load
remained undetectable. Perhaps this was a form of anxiety management.
Finally, when I asked Flor about the severity of her condition, she explained
that, "It's real serious—people *que estaban bien mal* [who were real sick]—I know
this dude that he got infected last year and it looked like he had been sick most
of his life . . . and he takes care of himself . . . [but] I don't think about that.
I don't think about bad things." Refusal to dwell on HIV helped Flor minimize
emotional paralysis and avoid feeling depression.

Of all of the women who spoke about the severity of their illness, Cristina
was the most ambivalent. She told me that her opinion changed daily. "It
depends. At times I think this is very serious, then at other times I just have this
'I don't care' attitude, you know. And I don't care, and that it doesn't bother me
whatever, and I just think it all depends on the mood I'm in [chuckles]."

Cristina described her on-again, off-again "devil-may-care" attitude, but
I never saw it. Whenever we spent time together, she talked of her illness with
an intensity tinged by fear. It almost seemed as though the weight of her worry
colored all of our interactions with tension and anxiety.

Visions of a Limited Future

A small group of women wondered how much time they had left. Nilsa fought a constant inner battle. Traumatized by symptoms, side effects, and the radical impact of the virus on her life, she found it difficult to remain optimistic in the face of her fears:

> I want to be an optimist. With the help of God I will be here a little longer, a good long time. But at times I think it won't happen—for example, when I feel ill. I feel sad, and I don't feel like I'm going to be here much longer.

Nilsa's Pentecostal faith kept her spirits up and pushed away the fear. She attended church at least twice a week, sometimes more often. Nilsa often told me that going to church helped her stay calm. It gave her something powerful and good to anchor her amidst the disorder of her life. This was true even though her minister called HIV/AIDS "a sinner's punishment from God." As a consequence, Nilsa kept her status a secret from all of her church friends but one. With this ally and her trust in God, she kept hopelessness at bay.

Gabrielle didn't think she'd be around much longer, either. "I think I got like four more years to live—'cause I can see my body deteriorating little by little. But I still got like four more years, with my ups and downs." Despite this sober assessment, she stayed actively engaged in her life and spent most of her days running errands with her granddaughter. Gabrielle also stayed actively involved with her treatment plan, consulting with her physician about all changes. Although she believed her time was limited, she wanted to make the most of it.

Cristina, who expressed such ambivalence about the severity of the illness, also thought her life was coming to a close. "I don't think I'll be around too long. I think I've had it long enough . . . well, I'm surprised I lasted this long. But I don't see myself living, two to three more years. No. No." Like Gabrielle, she worked hard to meet her goals in the time she had left. She had just regained custody of her adolescent son, and though he was not easy to care for, she was determined to give him a good life for as long as she could. But a tenacious syphilis co-infection, unsympathetic doctors, and recurrent bouts of addiction reinforced her belief that she would probably die sooner rather than later.

A few women did not even try to estimate the time they had left, but simply prayed that God would give them enough time to raise their children successfully—or at least until their children could take care of themselves. All women who had children at home identified this as a major source of anxiety. As Juana and Nini put it:

> I always think about my daughter, who is the only one. . . . I only ask that Jehovah gives me health and life, at least until my daughter can fight for herself on her own . . . at least until she is fifteen or sixteen years

old. . . . She is already a little bit grown. With all that one suffers, because my mother died six years ago now and I still suffer because of it. *Juana*

I don't know for how long. I ask God to give me more time. I have cancer and HIV—if not one, the other will kill me. I ask for an extension till Carlos is old enough to take care of himself. *Nini*

What Do You Fear Most about It?

Parenting Anxieties

The fear of being forced to abandon their children was the most pressing worry of the women I worked with. This is not surprising, since almost all were mothers with children still living at home. Many expressed a dread of not living to see their grandchildren:

Losing my kids. If it's going to happen, let it happen after my kids can make their own decisions. . . . [I want] nine more years . . . maybe fifty! [chuckles]. *Alicia*

What gets to me is my daughter. My daughter is the only thing [that bothers me]. The other thing, no, because after you die, you find rest. But, my daughter is the only thing I think about. *Juana*

Dying and leaving [her HIV-positive daughter]—leaving her here, you know. 'Cause I'm scared that they won't take care of her like they're supposed to. I prefer, see, to bury her first, and then I'll die. And then when I pass away, I'll pass away *tranquila*, at peace, no worry about nothing, you know. If anything I'm gonna be glad she's gonna be with me in the same hole and everything. *Flor*

I seem to have crying spells. Because I have five children . . . I know I'm not dying right now and I know I'm gonna last a long time. . . . But hey, I got kids, you know . . . everyone who has kids and has the virus and don't feel the way I feel don't have a heart, you know? *Selma*

Stigma and Fear of Becoming Grotesque

Two other common fears were usually mentioned together. The first was fear of a "worst-case AIDS death": wasting away in full view of family, friends, and neighbors, shrunken down to skeletal proportions. The second was to be stigmatized by such a visible AIDS death.

Well, what I fear the most is the, the disfigurement that people exhibit . . . when you can see all their bones, like that . . . because, if it's like this when I don't show any signs [of the illness], and now I know that often my family doesn't want to know anything about me, imagine [how they'll respond] when you can see [the signs of illness] in me! *Carlotta*

I don't think about my future—*hace mucho daño* [it does a lot of harm to do that]—but when I see people dying from AIDS, it's a reality and I can't ignore it. And I think it's painful seeing you—when I see myself in a bed all skinny, dying, and I'm afraid [for] my kids [and] grandkids [to see me]. *Nilsa*

Getting sick. Getting really, really sick. And looking like, you know. Like the last stages of AIDS. I think that's what frightens me the most. *Cristina*

Looking like that—real skinny, with a gray look. I'd rather die than have people feel sorry for me and treat me different. I'm afraid the people in here will find out, 'cause these people are very ignorant. I've been here twenty years, but [if the neighbors find out] I might have to move. That's what I'm afraid of. *Nini*

Getting sick and dying. Seeing my kids know. People in my family know[ing], and . . . how everyone reacts. *Selma*

When I see some of the people, like what they go through, like the wasting, and then the looking bad and the—skin lesions and people that I see with pneumonia, you know, difficult to breathe, oh my God. *Julia*

The worst imaginable future culminated in a bad death that left their children alone in the world. It was public death stamped with the telltale signs of AIDS. The women I worked with imagined that their loved ones would reject them once their secret could no longer be hidden. These anxieties were so common and so powerful that they emerged in our conversations again and again. It is likely that these fears were fanned by the exceptionally thin men and women who used the infectious disease clinics frequented by the women in my study. Sometimes, on clinic visits, the women I accompanied would point these skeletal folk out and whisper that they dreaded the thought of ever looking like them, a pattern that we will explore later.

Individual Fears

Some women mentioned other anxieties. Luchita, for example, feared the medicines more than she feared the disease itself. "The side effects of the medicines [scare me]. Why? Because the virus ain't gonna kill me . . . it's those medicines! The virus don't scare me, the side effects of the medicines scare me!" Although she tried to take several different drug combinations, they all caused severe side effects: nausea, extreme exhaustion, nightmares, and dizziness, among others. Luchita's frustration turned to disgust as she looked at her medication choices and concluded that they were all bad and just as likely to kill her as save her.

Celestina, who experienced nausea on all the HIV medications she had tried, also feared them.

Nerina, who traveled Newark and Elizabeth by bus, feared that the neuropathy that affected one of her legs might eventually confine her to a wheelchair. The thought chilled her to the bone. She left home almost every day to escape her abusive husband, who chased away visitors and friends. She had built her life around volunteering and socializing away from home. Anything that compromised her mobility would also cut her off from companions and decimate her coping strategy. "[I'm afraid of] the neuropathy. 'Cause I couldn't function without my legs. It would deprive me of, being with the people, you know? Going places, you know?"

What Are the Chief Problems It Causes?

Coping with Discrimination

The women I worked with answered me by describing the same problems again and again. Stigmatization and economic deprivation topped their list of problems. Whenever they entered a new environment, they worried about the possibility of rejection should their HIV-positive status be revealed. Many experienced the rejection of friends, family members, and lovers, which never ceased to cause them pain, even years later. Cristina spoke for several women when she explained that "The biggest problems . . . it has to do more with people than with myself. I have a lot of problems with relationships, friends. Family members—I have a feeling they don't even want me in their house." Several women stopped hugging relatives after the illness was revealed—not because they wanted to, but because they believed their touch was no longer welcome. As Gabrielle put it, "You can't be so close to people. You don't hug people. I mean in Puerto Rico. They are not educated [about HIV/AIDS]."

Those who had never disclosed their status worked hard to keep it secret. They felt their best protection was silence, at least among neighbors and distant family. But many told neither parents nor children. The constant vigilance required to maintain this position took an emotional toll. Nini described her struggle with this issue: "[The biggest problem is] making me lie to my kids, my mother, and my family. It changed my life completely."

Family members usually knew something was wrong. They asked about symptoms and frequent clinic visits. Women deflected attention with fabricated stories. But women's stories were often met with suspicion. Older children were especially likely to question their mothers. Alicia's teenagers loved to corner me and hammer out suspicious questions about their mother's health. Carlos, Nini's son, was very concerned about his mother's illness. His questions were so persistent that she finally told him the truth. But she made sure her mother and the rest of her family thought her cancer had recurred—which it later did, endangering her life but solidifying her story.

Even settings that should have been safe were often discriminatory. As Luchita observed, "When you go, like, to a clinic and tell them you're, like, HIV, they jump up like a chicken without a head, you know." She commented that physicians and nurses never expected her to have the virus; they reacted with shock when she told them. Julia, a veteran health advocate, commented acerbically that medical appointments and public meetings were excellent opportunities to experience prejudice.

Julia was not typical because she had once been very open about her status. She even appeared on a popular daytime talk show to talk about living with HIV. But over time, the repeated experience of discrimination wore her down. She became less and less willing to disclose her illness, until finally she stopped. When I asked her about the biggest problems caused by her illness, she told me why she and others like her had become less willing to talk about it.

> Being discriminated against, you know. Being cast aside . . . for example, I was admitted to a hospital one time and, and people were just making comments about people living with HIV there. That's why, a lot of times I don't even talk about it. . . . So, and I never like to be labeled; no matter what the situation is I never like that. I've noticed a lot of times when I go to a presentation or go do something that I'm knowledgeable, as soon as I say, "I'm HIV," right away like people see the fakeness on people's faces . . . and that's why a lot of people don't disclose a lot of times.

Economic Hardship and Household Management

Financial burdens caused nearly as many problems as discrimination. As the disease advanced, those who had worked either stopped, or lessened their participation in the formal and informal economy. "The informal economy" refers to income generation that is unregulated by legal economic institutions (Sharf 1998); in the United States, this is sometimes called working "under the table." For those who had derived their identity from work, it was a very difficult transition:

> It has caused me not to work now, which I loved going to work. And I can't work now for a year or something. It has caused trouble, trouble, trouble financially with the medicines that have to be paid and stuff. *Luchita*

The inability to work meant that households operated under constant financial strain. Children still had to be provided for; rent still had to be paid. The drugs used to treat HIV were prohibitively expensive, and women without Medicaid or ADAP (the AIDS Drug Assistance Program, designed to pay for the medications of uninsured or underinsured individuals) had to pay for their own. Even ADAP paid only for HIV-treatment drugs. Drugs for anything other than direct HIV care had to be paid for out of pocket.

Some women, like Paquita and Luchita, initially had neither Medicaid nor ADAP. These women used a variety of strategies to meet their expenses. Some took their children's leftover medicines when they were sick. Many depended on social service agencies to help pay utility and grocery bills. Most rented apartments under the HOPWA (Housing Opportunities for Persons with AIDS) program in order to find affordable housing. HOPWA offers housing subsidies to people living with HIV/AIDS and their families. Without a doubt, the most difficult economic challenge was finding and keeping a place to live. No matter what they did, the women I worked with could not provide their families with a financially secure lifestyle after their diagnosis.

When symptoms and opportunistic infections appeared or medication side effects emerged, things got even worse. Alicia, who spent most of her time and energy coping with chronic exhaustion and household chores, told me, "What I hate the most is not being able to be active with my kids." Sometimes the strain was so great that women questioned their own endurance. "I feel I can't keep going like this. I've been giving up, you know," said Nilsa. Her chronic headaches and continual search for safe, affordable housing created an almost untenable situation for her. She vacillated between rage and depression, wondering if she would be able to keep up her demanding round of clinic and physician visits while keeping her household together.

What Kinds of Treatments Do You Think You Should Receive?

Satisfaction with Standard Care

Given the serious nature of their problems and the many fears they faced, it was striking that at least six women were content with their medical care. Everyone wanted a cure, but quite a few were satisfied with their physicians. Some had excellent relationships with doctors who followed their care meticulously. These physicians acted almost like primary care physicians by embracing every aspect of their patients' care. They fostered healing relationships by entering into nonjudgmental, collaborative bonds with their patients and showing commitment to their care over time (Scott et al. 2008; Scott et al. 2009). Alicia, Julia, Nerina, and Nini all had relationships of this type, which will be explored further later on.

> I want a cure—that's what I want. I don't like . . . nobody likes to take medications. But for me it's working. And I'm pretty happy with this. *Alicia*

> I'm getting all the treatments so far. They treat me good. My doctor is waiting to give me HIV medication. If he waits, he can give me a better chance with one of the new ones when I really need it. *Nini*

But others who expressed positive feelings did not appear to receive high quality care. As I accompanied women to clinic appointments, I witnessed cursory physical exams, minimal physician investment, and care that was indifferent at best. I was surprised to find that some of the women who received this kind of care also expressed satisfaction. Both Carlotta and Selma fell into this group. After accompanying them on numerous clinic visits, I discovered they were lucky to get ten minutes of attention once a month, even when they were ill. I timed one of Carlotta's appointments at less than eight minutes, and Selma's consultations were only about three minutes longer. Some probing revealed that their satisfaction stemmed less from the quality of their care than from their lack of serious symptoms. They remained strong and functional with low viral load, and all of their symptoms were manageable.

> I'm content with the treatment that I have. Yes, I'm content because the medicines that I am taking have kept me strong and I know now how to keep it [the illness] under control. I know what I have to do at the moment and everything. I am well informed, so I think that the treatment I have is good. It works for me. *Carlotta*

> I'm satisfied with what I've got. I want a job. Beyond that I'm OK. *Selma*

Expanding Treatment Options

Other women were less satisfied and had strong opinions about how to improve their care. It was particularly common for them to focus on dissatisfaction with medications. Among the things they wanted was a once-a-day regimen with few side effects that required much less energy to manage properly (a once-a-day drug would not be available until 2006).

> A medication that helps people, but not killing you easily—that doesn't have so many side effects that affect people's bodies and that prolongs the life of a person a little bit. *Nilsa*

> I wish I could have something better than these medicines! *Luchita*

> Well, the cure. No, the truth is I don't know . . . at least all these pills you take together, if they could make them into just one. *Juana*

Some women wanted more access to nontraditional treatments. They wanted the opportunity to integrate complementary and alternative medicine, or CAM, therapies with more common medical treatments. Usually, they had been exposed to the herbal traditions of their grandparents or other older Latinos. Some had used CAM in the past or had been told of successful CAM use by HIV-positive men in their support groups or agency networks. These women wanted to use a wide range of options at the same time, often hoping to minimize medication side effects. Both women who expressed satisfaction with their medical care and those who were not as happy mentioned they'd like to use one or more CAM options.

> I want a homeopathic doctor to straighten my body out. And I used to do . . . that thing with the tapes . . . subliminal tapes. I wish I could get into that! I don't like drugs because they're too toxic, you know, dangerous! *Nerina*

> [I want] a mix of traditional and not so much toxic stuff, natural stuff. *Julia*

> Retreats for relaxation and stuff . . . like relaxing retreats. *Deborah*

> If the acupuncturist hadn't moved away, I'd still do that. *Alicia*

Almost all of these women were aware of several ways they could access CAM. Agencies ran no-cost retreats for men and women living with the virus, but waiting lists could be long. And at retreats and agency workshops, women encountered short introductions to everything from reiki to aromatherapy, t'ai chi, massage, and creative visualization. These experiences sometimes created a hunger to experience more. But it was often a challenge to maintain an ongoing relationship with an alternative therapist. Agency-sponsored sessions could lose funding, or therapists might work far away. Some therapies weren't available at all. Still, a surprising number of women managed to adopt one or more CAM modalities, either through self-care (by purchasing t'ai chi videos and using herbal supplements) or through government-funded programs for HIV support that offered acupuncture and massage. Sometimes practitioners were invited to support group meetings. However, the women I worked with wanted easier, more structured ways to incorporate CAM into their everyday treatment plans.

Emerging Patterns

All the women I worked with shared common experiences. At least half had been infected by husbands or trusted long-term partners. Almost all feared they would be forced to abandon their children due to a terrible wasting death. Most explained that their biggest problems did not come from the disease itself, but from medication side effects, discrimination, and the economic hardships that accompanied HIV. This is consistent with the findings of other researchers (Mosack et al. 2005).Yet many of these women—particularly those with broad cultural capital—believed they could live longer lives if they learned to manage the stresses they encountered every day. Their explanatory models prescribed the cultivation of inner calm, a daunting task for women facing HIV/AIDS and structural violence. It was striking, however, that none talked about gender relations as a source of risk. This is especially confounding because so many women told of contracting the virus from husbands and partners. This story, so common in Newark, was almost always perceived as a strictly personal tragedy.

Many women were satisfied with their medical care, although they were very unsatisfied with the drugs available to them. Based on my observations, this satisfaction came from the perception that the virus was under control rather than from the quality of care they received. Still, quite a few wanted to combine biomedical care with complementary and alternative options. They also hoped for a once-a-day drug without side effects. This falls in line with previous research showing that most HIV-positive individuals in developed nations use a combination of CAM and professional Western medicine (Sparber et al. 2000; Knippels and Weiss 2001; Standish et al. 2001; Gore-Felton et al. 2003).

However, there were important differences in explanatory models as well. While some women saw HIV as a curse (like Nini and Nilsa), two experienced it as a blessing (Gabrielle and Julia). This is similar to the findings of other studies exploring the perceptions and beliefs of HIV-positive individuals (Holmes and Pace 2002; Mosack et al. 2005). Some saw HIV as a wake-up call and an opportunity to reevaluate their life, while others associated it with serious physical and emotional loss. Finally, a few women offered structural or holistic perspectives on HIV rather than just providing personal explanations (Gabrielle, Selma).

Women who saw the virus as a predator or refused to name it (like Amelia, Nilsa, Carlotta, and Paquita) minimized their own agency and reported more ambivalence about the possibility of living a long, happy life. Women with average capital dominated this group. Those who saw themselves as active agents and attributed less power to the virus (like Nini, Deborah, Selma, Luchita, and Nerina) reported stronger beliefs that they could manage their health and live a long time. This group was made up of women with broad capital and women in the middle. All of these accounts underscore the need to respect the complexity of urban women's experiences and avoid minimizing either the challenges they face or the agency they retain. These findings also suggest that women's perceptions of their own agency help shape their visions of the future and their beliefs about what it may bring into their lives.

5

Managing Social Services

One day I arrived at Nini's house to find her stalking around the kitchen with an annoyed expression. "What's the matter?" I asked, as we flopped down at the kitchen table. "I just got off the phone with my case manager," Nini huffed. "She heard about a job and she wants me to call and apply right away. She's excited because it pays a little more than minimum wage and I've spent twenty minutes listening to her push me to call about it!"

"That's great!" I answered. "Maybe this will be a good thing and you can start working again." As a successful saleswoman, Nini had enjoyed a relatively high income in the past, selling mattresses, jewelry, and water filters. Now she found herself on welfare for the first time in her life and despised it. Though this mystery job would be no match for her top salary, I thought it might represent a good opportunity. But Nini literally snorted as she described the position: "This is a job with a florist. It would mean walking in and out of a freezer! I would be in the cold all day! How long do you think I would last if I took this job? My T-cell count is already low and I just got out of the hospital a few months ago. What do you think my immune system would do if I spent hours every day in a walk-in freezer?" "But why did the social worker even consider you for this job?" I asked. "Doesn't she know that you are HIV-positive?" "She knows," Nini replied crossly, "but she's ignorant. She just wants me to get off of welfare and she's not thinking about the risks."

Economic decisions have health consequences for everyone. Nini and her HIV-positive peers understood this very well. They weighed every financial decision for its possible health outcomes. The two domains were often so closely aligned for them that it was impossible to untangle economics from health; I noticed that financial brainstorming shaded into health management with great regularity.

The most basic economic decision was about how to make money. Almost everyone had children living at home and some also had husbands or long-term partners. Often women were both primary caregivers and breadwinners. They had to decide whether to continue working or apply for disability. When they did work, the money they made was rarely enough to meet their family's needs.

Like many HIV-positive individuals, Nini's career had been derailed by HIV disease and the depression that followed her diagnosis, but she was still the sole provider for herself and her teenage son. When we met, her finances were strained as she struggled to pay her monthly telephone and energy bills. Even small expenses were a major challenge. Because Nini had always worked and was accustomed to a middle-class standard of living, she defined herself through her career. The drastic drop in income she now faced enraged her. But although Nini was always searching for ways to make more money, she had been forced to accept the fact that many job opportunities would do her more harm than good. Despite her quest for a steady income, her primary consideration had to be the preservation of her immune system; after all, she hoped to raise her son to adulthood.

Our kitchen conversation about how to address the money problem mirrored community debates everywhere. In clinic waiting rooms all over Newark, HIV-positive patients occupied themselves by comparing the health impact of regular employment with that of filing for disability. Conventional wisdom said that those who worked died sooner than those who filed. If you did not stop working once you became symptomatic, you were in trouble. And few unskilled workers were excited about risking their lives to keep the minimum-wage jobs available to them. But work had its benefits as well as its drawbacks. Some people didn't want to stop for fear of getting bored or losing their identity; others didn't want to lose control of their money. Celestina, for example, no longer worked for pay, but this was not by choice. One day as we walked by a fast food restaurant, she murmured sadly in Spanish, "I miss Burger King. Did you know that I worked there for more than ten years? If I could, I would still work there." Luchita, too, missed her role as a home health aid. When medication side effects compelled her to stop working, she spoke of it as a loss, as noted in chapter 2.

Applying for Disability

The two disability programs to which Nini could have applied were SSDI (Social Security Disability Insurance) and SSI (Supplemental Security Income). However, applying to either program did not guarantee success. When Nini realized that she could no longer work full time, she applied for disability under the SSDI program. She chose this option because she had worked for many years and she knew that the amount of her monthly check would be based on her prior earnings record as well as the social security taxes she had paid into the system. Since she had worked all her life, she thought her benefits would be considerable.

To apply, Nini submitted her claim to the New Jersey Disability Determination Services (DDS) office. She included medical and mental health records from doctors, therapists, clinics, and caseworkers. She also included a printout of all her medications. To prove that she had worked for long enough to qualify, she listed the names and addresses of all her employers, beginning in 1985. Unfortunately, this was not enough. Her symptoms did not match those on the official list of HIV-related opportunistic infections (OIs) used by DDS, and her claim was denied. Disability benefits were granted based on the presence of these OIs, and though the list had been revised in 1993 in order to better include women's complaints, female applicants were still denied more frequently than men (Kurth 1993). Nini tried again a year later and was denied a second time, so she visited an aide at a local free legal clinic, who explained that it would be difficult for her to win an appeal because she was a woman. When she heard this, she began preparing as if she were going to war, even consulting a Santera (a priestess of Santeria) for help. "The lady at the clinic is real good, but hello! I'm not taking any chances. I'm going to kill a chicken for it," she said, referring to the ceremony she was about to commission.

Because Nini faced a deeply entrenched institutionalized gender bias, the aide advised her to submit a letter of support from her psychiatrist emphasizing her mental health diagnosis. This, she felt, would strengthen Nini's case. At her following psychiatric visit, Nini explained the situation and her psychiatrist agreed to write a letter supporting her appeal. Nini showed me his letter, in which he asked DDS to approve her claim based on a diagnosis of major depression. "Her depression has worsened due to intrinsic and extrinsic circumstances. Her concentration dwindles after ten minutes. Her attention span fluctuates and her short-term memory is impaired. Emotionally she is not able to withstand the usual stresses of a regular gainful job. Based on all these findings, I urge you to consider to provide this patient with all the support your agency is capable of" (Field letter excerpt 1997). This time, her appeal was successful. Afterward, Nini and her aide agreed that she had won because her case had hinged on depression rather than HIV.

Both Nini's ex-sister-in-law Flor and her friend Nilsa applied for disability through SSI, the Supplemental Security Income program. Neither had spent sufficient time in the workforce to qualify for Social Security Disability Insurance. The two women also submitted their medical records to the New Jersey Disability Determination Services office. Unlike her, they were required to document their poverty, showing little or no access to income or economic resources. Compared to SSDI benefits, the SSI checks they received were tiny. Even after the state of New Jersey added an additional contribution to the national SSI allowance, the maximum 1997 monthly payment for those living alone was only $515.25 a month. For someone living with an ineligible spouse it was slightly higher—$751.36 (SSA 1995a; SSA 1995b; SSA 1997). Living on this amount was tremendously challenging for the successful applicant. Luckily, most SSI recipients were also eligible for food stamps (SSA 1997). Both Flor and Nilsa succeeded in their applications and were awarded SSI benefits with food stamps; Nilsa, whose son who was cognitively disabled, was able to get a monthly SSI check for him as well.

Perhaps the most important difference between SSI (Flor and Nilsa's program) and SSDI (Nini's program) was the striking difference in medical insurance offered through each one (SSA n.d.). Once an individual qualified for SSI, all potentially qualifying members of that person's household were automatically enrolled in Medicaid, the nation's medical insurance program for those living below the poverty level (SSA 1995a; SSA 1995b; SSA 1997). For women living with HIV, this was extremely important. Because they could become seriously ill at any time, medical insurance was as important as a monthly check. But SSDI did not offer automatic Medicaid eligibility. After two years, SSDI beneficiaries qualified for Medicare, the nation's supplemental insurance program for the elderly (SSA 1995a; SSA 1995b). During their first two years, however, successful SSDI applicants like Nini had to find some other way to pay for their health care. Some depended on private insurance, but most did not have this option. They simply cobbled together whatever resources they could assemble and did the best they could. After two years, SSDI's Medicare benefits kicked in, and although they were superior to SSI's Medicaid benefits, the unlucky died waiting for them.

There was one loophole: very low-income persons with a qualifying work history could qualify for both SSDI and SSI. These individuals could enroll in Medicaid through SSI and later qualify for Medicare through SSDI (SSA 1995a; SSA 1995b; SSA 1997; SSA n.d.). But the women in my study found it challenging enough to apply for one program, much less two. Most did not even know that it was possible to apply for both. Only Nerina and Nini applied for both SSDI and SSI. Both had extensive work histories and broad cultural- and social-capital toolkits.

The Stigma of Welfare

After Nini's first SSDI claim was denied, she needed another strategy for securing a steady income. Sick or not, she needed money to raise her son and run her household. Nini decided to apply for welfare benefits, but she was angry about it. Had HIV passed her by, she would never have been pushed into this course of action. "I've never been on welfare!" she raged. "I have always taken care of myself and my children. I hate this!" In addition to adding to her depression, welfare was a temporary solution at best.

In the mid-1990s federal welfare reform was the subject of great debate; Congress passed a series of laws ushering in "work fare," programs designed to transition welfare recipients into the paid workforce (Zippay and Rangarajan 2005). New Jersey's welfare initiative, the "Work First New Jersey" program, went into effect on July 1, 1997. Those receiving benefits were notified of the new work activity requirements: they would now have to participate in job training and take a volunteer position or engage in some other approved activity. Failure to enroll in an approved Work First activity meant that their welfare case would be terminated in ninety days, eliminating both cash benefits and Medicaid eligibility. Furthermore, the new regulations put a five-year cap on the length of time they could collect assistance (Zippay and Rangarajan 2005).

This change impacted many of New Jersey's HIV-positive women, including Nini and Deborah. Deborah was eager to transition from a volunteer to a paid position, but she worried about keeping her health care benefits: "For Work First, I'm volunteering to keep my Medicaid benefits. So I go to school [a job-training program] on Monday from nine to three, I volunteer at the hospital, on Tuesday from nine to three, Wednesday I'm at school again, and Thursday and Friday I'm at the hospital all day. . . . If I find a part-time job, like at five dollars an hour, automatically they'll cut off my food stamps and money, but they'll leave me with Medicaid. I get $424 a month [and] $100 in food stamps for me, my daughter, and my daughter's baby. If I get [a job that pays] seven dollars an hour, they'll cut me off completely—off of Medicaid! I would be working to pay for my medications."

Nini received a Work First notification letter from Newark's Division of Welfare while she was waiting to appeal her SSDI denials. The letter explained that she was required to appear for an interview with a new Work First case manager in a week and a half or lose her welfare benefits. Despite this development, Nini decided to focus on moving her SSDI appeal forward rather than trying to find a (paid or volunteer) position compatible with her compromised state of health. Her persistence paid off when she won, and her welfare benefits were replaced with SSDI and eventually SSI.

The Problem of Housing

Even with SSDI benefits, Nini's money problems remained unresolved. Like many other urban single mothers, she found that SSDI/SSI did not provide enough income to support her family (Sharff 1998). Those of her peers who continued working couldn't take care of their families either. So almost all of them turned to HOPWA, the Housing Opportunities for Persons with HIV/AIDS program. Established in 1992 by the Department of Housing and Urban Development, HOPWA was designed to meet the housing needs of low-income people living with HIV/AIDS and their families (HUD). Newark is exactly the type of urban setting in which HOPWA can help level the playing field for people with HIV. The city's chronic shortage of affordable housing makes competition for decent apartments fierce. Before HOPWA, HIV-positive individuals looking for a place to live could be at a serious disadvantage.

HOPWA funds can be used for housing, social service program planning, and development projects. Not-for-profit organizations can use them to buy, build, or rehabilitate houses and apartments intended for HIV-positive people and their families or use HOPWA funds to place individuals in SROs—single-occupancy hotel rooms (HUD). Women usually apply for long-term rental assistance through HOPWA so they can rent apartments on the private market. They generally discover the program through a case manager at a social service agency who can document their HIV status and low income, helping them apply. I observed that the process was not easy: waiting lists were long and apartments hard to find, but the women in my study depended on HOPWA because it paid for both the security deposit and up to 70 percent of an apartment's monthly rent (HUD).

When HOPWA applicants finally reached the top of the waiting list they had to find an apartment that met program standards. Apartments were required to have a living room, a kitchen, and a bathroom as well as one sleeping area for every two family members. Each room had its own separate requirements and every apartment had to pass an official inspection. Finally, the rent had to fall within the HUD Fair Market Rent Index for its geographic area (HUD). Finding an apartment that met all of these standards was difficult. Women with broad social capital turned to friends and acquaintances to ease the challenge. Julia explained it like this:

> My landlord is a friend, and he takes HOPWA, which pays three-quarters of the rent and I pay one-quarter. He's a real friend, but I don't know if the next landlord will take it. I can only live in this nice place because of HOPWA. Not everyone takes it because they always pay late. They always pay late and they don't want to pay any late fees either. So landlords get angry unless you have the money to pay one month ahead, plus down payment. How can they accept this? Most Newark landlords don't. Deborah's landlord went right up and knocked on her door and yelled, "When am I gonna get my rent?" so that everybody could hear. So people don't have much choice about where they live. Nobody can pay a month in advance.

Nini wanted an apartment in a good neighborhood that also met HUD's criteria. Like Julia, she used her vast social network to locate a decent apartment with a sympathetic landlord. Her HOPWA-approved rental contract covered the security deposit and paid $500 of her $625 rent, leaving her responsible for the remaining $125. This was a great price for a two-bedroom Newark apartment, and Nini was delighted with her results: a safe, low-cost apartment in a pleasant neighborhood.

But for women with average capital, the same search could turn into a nightmare. Without a large social network, it could be nearly impossible to find a safe, qualifying apartment. Both Cristina and Nilsa struggled with this problem. In New Brunswick, a city twenty-eight miles away, Cristina was looking for a two-bedroom apartment that would pass inspection and rent at HUD's index price. Unlike Julia and Nini, she had little social capital and couldn't find any help. To make matters worse, her search put her in direct competition with Rutgers undergraduates looking for cheap off-campus housing. In combination with HUD's high safety standards and the $929 price cap for the area, this meant that Cristina could not find a place.

As time passed, she became more and more desperate: without a qualifying two-bedroom apartment she couldn't obtain custody of her son. After several months, the stress pushed her into relapse. "I'm kind of embarrassed to tell you, but when I didn't call you back, I was using. The stress got so bad that I went back to it for a little while. Every apartment I found had something wrong with it," she explained. When she found an apartment that passed inspection, she stopped using drugs, but the whole experience left her depressed and spent.

Working the Agencies

Government programs like SSDI, SSI, and HOPWA were not the only important sources of help for women. Alliances with not-for-profit social service agencies were also critical. They referred their clients to important programs like HOPWA and provided families with resources they could not normally afford. Ideally, agency staff workers knew the full range of programs available in an area and some were willing to share this knowledge. Each agency specialized in solving one or more of the problems likely to plague HIV-positive women and their families: how to pay larger-than-expected utility bills, how to get an air conditioner during a long, hot summer, and how to find a free therapist capable of counseling anxious children. Relationships with agency workers and volunteers could mean access to free groceries, clothes, toys, medications, medical care, complementary and alternative medicine (CAM), transportation, and furniture, as well as a host of other resources.

Women with a broad cultural-capital toolkit used it to build alliances with agency workers in order to access benefits of this kind. For a family surviving on disability and food stamps, these benefits could mean the difference between a reasonable life and a tragic one. As women with broad capital explored agency resources, they asked themselves a series of questions. How many agencies lie within a reasonable distance and what does each have to offer? How are they organized? What kinds of problems could I encounter there? A good working knowledge of agency funding was an asset in answering them all. The most successful alliance builders I met gathered as much information as they could by talking to each other and agency staff whenever possible. They also offered this knowledge to others in need of help. I will explore the significance of these questions through field note excerpts and direct quotes. All agency names are pseudonyms.

How Many Local Agencies Lie within a Reasonable Distance and What Does Each Have to Offer?

One day Nini introduced me to Teresa, a newly diagnosed Puerto Rican woman whom she had recently met. As we settled into Nini's kitchen, she began educating Teresa about agency resources in her area. First, she told Teresa about an AYUDA (pseudonym for a local social service agency) program that offered each client a large bag of groceries once a month. Although their dollar value was low, each bag included the most critical staples used by Latino families: rice, beans, jars of recaito (a cilantro-based seasoning), and other cooking basics. Just as importantly, the food was delivered by social workers making home visits so Teresa didn't need a car to pick it up.

Nini also told Teresa that other area agencies also offered their clients groceries, but they were either culturally inappropriate or required that families pick them up themselves. This usually meant hiring an expensive taxi or committing the time to an uncomfortable bus ride. Nini pointed out that there was no point in going to an agency that did either of those things when an easier, better option was available. For a woman managing medication side effects or HIV-related symptoms, the energy saved could be especially valuable. "AYUDA and Helping Hands [another agency pseudonym] provide food vouchers and bags of food, and if they have to bring it to a person's house, they bring it there. Those are the only two agencies that provide any useful [groceries]," Nini explained.

It might have taken Teresa weeks or even months to discover this on her own. Had she felt nervous about venturing into the AIDS community, she might never have learned it at all. In the absence of expert guidance, many of the women I met had to figure out what *not* to do through frustrating rounds of trial and error.

Knowing the details of each local program helped women overcome adversity and assist others to do so. Like Nini, Julia spent a great deal of time educating peers about local resources. As a caseworker at a small agency, she was especially knowledgeable about what was locally available. Deborah told me the story of how Julia helped her transition from homelessness to an affordable apartment in which she could live with her daughter:

> Somebody introduced [Julia] to me and I was telling her about my problems and she gave me her card and I called her. I went in to speak to her.

And she told me that I didn't have to live like that. So she told me to go to the welfare office and apply for welfare for my daughter, get custody of my daughter first, which was easy because my daughter had the willingness to come back home with me. And I got temporary custody of my son, every other weekend, so I went to Julia, she was my social worker, she got me in touch with programs that they had. And she told me to get a written receipt and they paid for my light and my gas to turn it on, and that's how I got my apartment.

How Are My Local Agencies Organized?

Paying attention to an agency's size, target audience, and organizational culture was also valuable. Successful alliance builders quickly learned that larger agencies offered a range of non-HIV-related programs and this meant more potential resources. Smaller agencies were usually more focused on HIV-related work, but their staff often had more direct experience with the challenges of living with HIV/AIDS. Tiny agencies and departments offered the fewest programs but the most personal attention and individualized support. By understanding how each agency was organized and run, a woman could choose the kind of services she preferred.

It was also useful to know who had founded each agency and what groups they had originally intended to serve. Some had been created by particular cultural or religious groups and operated primarily within their own communities. AYUDA and ASISTENCIA (both pseudonyms), for example, served mostly Spanish-speaking clients. Project Connect, however, served predominantly African American clients. Crossing cultural and religious lines was a useful strategy for women attempting to broaden their social networks, but women with average capital almost always felt more comfortable with agencies created from within their own *habitus.*

What Problems Could I Encounter?

Once women knew where to go for the programs they needed and understood how their local agencies were organized, they had to master one more task: how to recognize and address potential conflicts of interest. According to Nini, "HIV agencies are interested in getting money for themselves. They take our money—money that was set aside for us—and they use it [for] themselves." This seemed to be a harsh assessment, but as I spent more time with the women of Newark and Elizabeth, I began to understand why she and some of her peers felt this way. Over time, I noticed that institutional needs sometimes eclipsed the needs of individual clients. This didn't mean that agencies were unhelpful, nor that their intentions weren't good; it simply meant that their desire to help was balanced—and occasionally superseded—by the desire to protect their own viability.

All of the most successful alliance builders in my study collected information about potential conflicts of interest as they frequented each organization. Nini, Julia, and Deborah were the most adept practitioners of this strategy. They used multiple agency programs concurrently and referred their peers to those that they knew about but did not use. They consciously assessed each organization they encountered, paying close attention to everything they saw and heard for their own benefit and that of their friends. Julia explained it this way: "You just have to sit down and ask and ask, and then you get this answer from this social worker, and another from an intake person, and the other one from the agency director . . . and then you see what you need to do."

One example of a conflict of interest involved social security numbers and their role in client-consultation reimbursement. "We are numbers to them," Nini explained to Carlotta. "[Agencies] always want that little number." Early on, she discovered that the single largest HIV funding source, the Ryan White Comprehensive AIDS Resources Emergency (CARE) Act, required social service agencies to confirm the citizenship and eligibility of each client through social security numbers (HRSA; HRSA 2006).

Then and now, most HIV-focused agencies depend on Ryan White funding. The CARE act was ratified in 1990 and named for the famous Indiana teenager whose struggle with discrimination made AIDS-related stigma a national issue. The act funds a wide range of primary health care and support services for those living with HIV. As the largest single source of HIV care and service funding in this country, it has been critical in shaping and sustaining HIV/AIDS-related services (HRSA).

The Fifteen-Minute Rule

During my fieldwork, agency staff explained that organizations dependant on Ryan White funding were usually reimbursed for their services based on a formula allotting fifteen minutes per client consultation. Essentially, this meant that agencies were reimbursed for only the first fifteen minutes of any consultation. I was told that the fifteen-minute formula imposed a hardship on case managers and clients alike: frustrated social workers complained that fifteen minutes was too short a time in which to clarify most clients' problems, much less resolve them. Some case managers were expected to identify clients' issues, develop action plans, and make referrals in that time—a process that could barely be started in fifteen minutes. Under this system, the most financially rewarding kind of contact was a phone call! One overstressed case manager explained that social workers were often caught between clients who needed more time and administrators who wanted them to bill for more consultations.

This worker explained that smaller agencies were less likely to emphasize the fifteen-minute rule. He explained that modest programs and sparser settings usually offered social workers more freedom to judge the amount of time needed to help each client as well as the freedom to adjust their schedules accordingly. "It's not what you would think, but a small agency with less funding can be more effective than a large one with more money." He pointed out that investing greater care and attention on fewer clients resulted in fewer reimbursements but better client outcomes.

Awareness of the fifteen-minute rule could help women prepare for potential challenges and respond more effectively when they occurred. A client with a serious problem could wait a long time in exchange for fifteen minutes with an overwhelmed caseworker. If that worker was forced to follow the rule, she or he might be more likely to resist listening to the whole story. Or the worker might decide to address the narrowest slice of the problem. It could also mean that the caseworker might throw the ball right back into the client's lap as soon as possible. Most commonly, this manifested as the following chant: "Before we can do anything, you need to bring in X paperwork, a bill showing your name and address, and a current ID."

"Guarding" Clients

Another agency staff member explained a second practice that women frequently encountered. Since agency reimbursement was based on the total number of client contacts as evidenced by social security numbers, each client was a valuable resource. Losing a client to another agency or even sharing a client could mean loss of funding. In some agencies, workers were encouraged to make sure that clients stayed "in-house" by keeping all referrals within the agency or its parent institution. Clients were shuffled back and forth among different subsidiary departments in order to keep Ryan White money in the same organization. This strategy helped agencies stay solvent but sometimes had a negative impact on women looking for help.

Imagine that Remedios, a client of Agency A, visits her case manager about a phone bill she cannot pay. Her case manager knows that Agency A does not have Ryan White money earmarked for emergency telephone bill payments. They only offer HIV support groups, referrals to an affiliated hospital ID clinic, and health care education. But the case manager knows that Agency B *does* have a telephone bill program. Yet she doesn't tell Remedios that she can probably get the bill paid if she goes to Agency B. In theory, the case manager could even phone Agency B to speed up the process, but what if Remedios never comes back to Agency A? Even if the case manager really wants to help, her job could be at risk if she refers Remedios out of the organization. It may be easier and safer for the case manager to explain that she can do nothing in this case. If Remedios does not know much about local agencies or understand the conflicts of interest possible under Ryan White funding, she might accept what she is told and go away.

The Ryan White CARE Act

Sometimes case managers didn't know about other programs; with so many agencies and a constantly changing menu of programs, information quickly goes out of date. Because of this and because the Ryan White CARE Act structures the distribution of so many resources, it is important that everyone with a stake in HIV/AIDS care understand how the system works. Ryan White funds are divided into different funding pools referred to as "Titles." Many social service support programs are funded with Title I money, and the more HIV-related services and programs each institution offers, the more it depends on Ryan White Title I money to survive. For example, HIV-focused agencies like Renewal (a pseudonym) used Ryan White funds to support most of their work, while organizations with only a few HIV-related programs applied for smaller amounts of Title I grant money (HRSA; NEMA Planning Council; HRSA 2006).

Title I funding also has another relevant feature: it channels its dollars to grant recipients through geographic regions called "EMAs" or "Eligible Metropolitan Areas." An EMA is a somewhat flexible geographic construct created to define an area heavily impacted by HIV/AIDS. Newark's EMA is referred to as "NEMA" (Newark Eligible Metropolitan Area). It includes Essex, Morris, Sussex, Union, and Warren counties (NEMA Planning Council; HRSA 2006). In order to receive and redistribute Ryan White Title I funds, each EMA must create its own EMA planning council, and NEMA is no different. The NEMA Planning Council includes both PWAs who receive services and HIV service providers, because federal rules mandate that local people living with the virus make up a significant proportion of the group.

HIV planning councils must include a diverse group of HIV-positive individuals, including service providers, health care professionals, and PWAs from local communities of color. The planning council determines how Title I funds will be distributed within its EMA. While it is the intent of the Ryan White CARE Act that local clients and providers collaborate to decide where the bulk of NEMA's Title I money goes (NEMA Planning Council), they do not always agree. Recall that chapter 3 describes the 1992–1993 planning council power struggle that resulted in Newark's loss of millions in Ryan White funding (Wilson 1992). Berger's study of HIV-positive women in Detroit also noted that the interests of different planning council groups do not always coincide (Berger 2004).

I found that agency staff with the most comprehensive grasp of NEMA's programs worked at the local HIV consortium. HIV consortia exist to coordinate service-delivery efforts across EMAs; they act in conjunction with planning councils to channel Title I funds. The Union County HIV Consortium Resource Center, part of the NEMA Planning Council, describes its mission this way:

> . . . to develop a coordinated plan to respond to the HIV epidemic as it
> occurs in Union County; provide a forum for agencies that provide services

to persons who are HIV-positive and/or have HIV disease in order that services may be coordinated, developed, enhanced and improved; maximize existing resources and stimulate program development according to the needs of the HIV-positive population; serve as a conduit to recipient agencies or groups; seek funding from public or private bodies in order to advance the mission; provide technical assistance concerning provision of services to member organizations; educate and enhance community awareness; act as a clearinghouse and resource center for members and the general public concerning the HIV epidemic. (Union County HIV Consortium n.d.)

The Union County HIV Consortium has approximately fifty-three member agencies, sixteen individual members, and five associate member agencies, and its "membership represents provider agencies, advocates, the affected population and interested individuals." Because of this, its staff were often in the best possible position to understand the program universe as it existed across NEMA and match people with the programs they needed (NEMA Planning Council). Ironically, because the consortium focused on coordination *across* agencies rather than on generating its own programs, it often struggled to get its own Ryan White funding. This created an absurd situation in which the least biased organization had the most difficulty surviving.

Agency Barriers: Competition and Conflicts of Interest

The most successful alliance builders I met understood that the interests of HIV-positive individuals and the agencies that served them were not always the same. They quickly grasped that since all NEMA agencies depended on more or less the same Ryan White funding, they were all, at some level, in competition with each other. Nini summarized it like this: "That's what makes me angry, OK? Because a lot of people don't see us like, like persons, they just see us like money and that really upsets me because any time that I go to speak to a social worker that's all they care about . . . the money they are going to get. The first thing they ask for is the last four digits of your social security number!"

Agencies that served the same communities found themselves in even closer competition. They were often evaluated against each other by clients held in common. In one major geographic area, at least four different agencies targeted Latino clients. One specialized in meeting the needs of older adults and another concentrated on a small group of neighborhoods. The two remaining agencies offered a range of HIV-related programs to an overlapping group of clients. Each had its own area of expertise. The smaller of the two employed a tiny group of case managers to serve its HIV-positive clients.

This department benefited from its size in that its workers had plenty of opportunities to get to know clients personally, but it suffered in that it offered a limited menu of services. Case managers developed close relationships with each family during the course of household visits, and they were also able to consider each client's needs on an individualized basis. I never heard a negative evaluation of this agency's performance in all the years I spent in the field. No one complained to me about them, even though they had few programmatic offerings.

The larger of the two agencies provided a wider range of services, employed more workers, and was better known throughout the community. It probably took in significantly more Ryan White money than its smaller counterpart. This organization seemed to have a more turbulent relationship with its clients than its diminutive peer, and I heard periodic complaints about its employees and services. If one were to judge solely by size, range of services, and level of funding, this agency would seem more successful, yet clients of both organizations in my small sample did not seem to feel this way.

Nini contrasted the two organizations like this:

> It's a big rip-off. [The small one] is the only agency that comes to your house if you are sick—if you need a ride to go to your doctor, they take you to the doctor, they wait for you, they bring you home. They are the only agency that will help you after hours. But [the larger one] doesn't provide transportation even for people who are really sick, OK? Hello, they got vans, but they don't want to use it. They use it for their own purposes, to go to meetings. If they want to go to a meeting, they can manage themselves! People need it more to go to the doctor, to social security, or to welfare! [The small agency] goes out of their way, and not just for me—for every single client. Their counselors go pick people up from the street that have been going back in drugs and take them to the hospital. They make sure they stay in the hospital and bring them back to the program. I have seen that from [the small agency] and it's getting less money than [the larger one], OK?

Nilsa's struggle to get housing demonstrates how easily clients could get caught between competing agencies. When I met her, she spent an inordinate amount of time searching for a better apartment. She and her son rented a two-bedroom apartment in a housing project near Nini's neighborhood. Financially, it was a good deal because the apartment was subsidized through HOPWA's rental assistance program. However, it was located in an ugly, run-down area, overrun with drug dealers who ran their businesses out of buildings flanking Nilsa's. One day I surprised one of them hiding drugs in a hole next to Nilsa's door. Nilsa hated her apartment for all of these reasons, but especially because of what she feared for her oldest son. He had been put in a facility for teenage offenders on drug-related charges. He had been away for a year when I met her. Nilsa worried that when he returned, the drug-saturated environment would lead him directly back to where he started. Although she did not have strong relationships with any particular agency or case manager, Nilsa began visiting agency after agency in order to find help locating a HOPWA-subsidized, drug-free place to live. "I have to find another place," she told me. "This one is disgusting . . . the police come and they [the drug dealers] are gone for one week, two weeks. Then the police go and they come back. But no one will listen to me. 'You've already got a place,' they say. 'We can't help you.' But I can't stay here."

Nini suggested that Nilsa visit the larger Latino social service agency to ask for help. Nini had heard that this agency had access to subsidized apartments in a better neighborhood. Nilsa described her visit to a case worker there. After completing her intake forms she explained her problem. "Have you been to any other agencies?" asked the case worker. Nilsa replied that she sometimes visited them, but that none had been able to help her find an apartment in a safer neighborhood. The worker used Nilsa's social security number to access her records on a NEMA-wide social service data system, and then turned to face Nilsa again. "You went to [the small social service agency] last month to pick up groceries," she said. "I'm sorry, we can't help you." Nilsa pressed her, probing for any relevant programs for which she might qualify. The worker stood firm, repeating "We can do nothing for you." The conversation became more heated until the case manager picked up Nilsa's intake forms and tore them in half. Shocked, Nilsa retreated, ready to give up.

When Nini learned about the incident she pressed Nilsa to protest what had happened. After repeated urging, Nilsa finally asked me to help her write a letter of complaint about the incident. We sent copies to the case worker, her supervisor, and the director of the agency, but Nilsa never received a response. The experience demoralized her and filled her with rage at her own powerlessness. "I can't do nothing about it," she said bitterly when I asked her if she had heard anything about a new apartment.

Women with average capital were more likely to express feelings of intimidation when discussing their relationships with the agencies they frequented. Most understood that Ryan White funds had been set aside by the government to help them and they felt entitled to a certain amount of that help. But when they reached out for it, they often encountered barriers that made the process seem too difficult to pursue. They wanted a help-seeking process that did not generate any new burdens to add to those they already had. If too many trips, forms, check stubs, or stressful conversations were required, it was easier to just live with the original problem.

A lot of days I want to move, to get a better apartment. Not in this neighborhood. But I can't. I pay $97 in rent [a month] after HOPWA pays. And now my rent is going up $25 to $550. When I see the social worker at [a social service agency], they're just gonna make me pay more rent. *Amelia*

"Why don't more people complain?" I asked Nini after an afternoon of horror stories. "Because they are afraid!" she retorted. "They think that if they complain, they won't get any help at all, so they keep their mouths shut. They need every little bit—they can't afford to be turned away." Nini did not feel this way. She complained both to me and to the staff of agencies that annoyed her. Her vast social network protected her because it gave her the ability to publicly shame those who offended her. "They're afraid of me!" she exclaimed. "They know I have a big mouth." Nini's critical eye missed nothing, and over time, she accumulated quite a bit of knowledge about how agencies operated.

OK, every time that each one of us goes [to an agency], it gets $72. Look, if they have a social worker there they get $75. Where does the money go? Take Agency Q [a pseudonym]. They get $75 a visit there, but you're only gonna get $100 a year from them if you need help paying your PSE&G bill. They don't help you pay your telephone bill or get food vouchers. . . . At the moment [this agency] is just for prevention. It's not a place that you can get help if you are already HIV-positive. They don't have much to offer, so they try to do a support group.

Conflicts of interest emerged in other ways as well. When working with organizations that served both HIV-positive and HIV-negative groups, women worried that their HIV-negative neighbors might see them and guess their status. Caridad and Nini each avoided at least one agency for this reason. One day, a volunteer at one of these organizations asked Caridad why she visited the agency so often.

She was the one who filled out the papers . . . and then she said, "So, why do you come here so often?" That's a lack of respect. Why should she ask me what I am doing there? That's not her problem . . . so I didn't go back.

The issue was different when working with HIV-focused agencies. Most ran support groups in which members and facilitators were instructed to keep everything confidential. If one could arrive without being seen, it was possible to keep one's status a secret. But group facilitators did not always succeed at keeping discussions private. Nini told me about one such experience: "It was a very close group. The things we said used to stay behind those walls. But then, the people who worked there started talking. Everything was out in the street. I used to pick up my phone and hear, 'Oh! She said this about you.' So I stopped going." Breaches of confidentiality are serious transgressions with potential legal consequences, and although agencies worked hard to prevent them, they were not always successful.

Emerging Patterns

Regardless of how women viewed government programs and social service organizations, they acknowledged that they were crucial resources. Every woman who worked with me had at least one neutral relationship with a social service agency and most tried to cultivate more than one.

Women with average capital had greater social support needs than their broad capital counterparts, but they were often unable to get the help they needed. Although they tried to establish good relationships with agency workers, they frequently failed. Cristina, Nilsa, and Amelia struggled to find help throughout the length of my study. All three needed help finding safe, affordable housing but didn't get it.

Although each woman eventually found someplace to live, none could thrive in the apartments they found. Nilsa's greatest fears were realized when her son returned to her drug- and violence-infested housing project and began using again. The stress of Cristina's apartment search contributed to her return to drugs. Amelia didn't even try to find a better apartment for another year, and when her family finally did move, their new building stood next to an abandoned house used by prostitutes. While six of the eight women with broad capital (Deborah, Julia, Nerina, Nini, Selma, and Caridad) and one of the two women in the middle (Alicia) were successful at creating strong social service alliances, only one woman with average capital (Flor) was able to do so.

Women with broad capital used it to gather information about what was available, how agencies were structured, and what conflicts might emerge; they were very successful at building alliances with multiple organizations. When these women encountered organizational barriers, they used their knowledge to circumvent or confront or them. When they could not bend a system enough to make it useful, they moved on to other agencies and options.

Nini, Julia, and Deborah all set up patterns of reciprocity with their social service allies, sending them new clients and attending unpopular workshops to

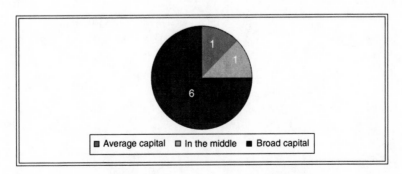

| ▣ Average capital | ▢ In the middle | ▪ Broad capital |

FIGURE 5.1 Strong Social Service Alliances

get attendance up. They brought their HIV-positive friends to agency programs to teach them about local resources while helping their allies keep the grant money that kept them in business. In return, they were the first to be called whenever new resources became available: clothes, groceries, or free air conditioners. Their refrigerators were packed with turkeys at Thanksgiving and their pantries were often stocked with free groceries. All of these women acted as redistribution centers, giving much of what they got to needier HIV-positive friends and acquaintances without the social capital to get them on their own.

Despite the fact that every woman in my study needed the support of government programs and social service agencies, women with average capital and women with broad capital developed very different relationships with them. This suggests that a range of outreach and retention strategies are needed in order to ensure that those women who need help the most actually receive it.

6

Working the Clinics

"Pastillas y No Explicaciones" (Pills, Not Explanations)

One sunny afternoon I stopped at Carlotta's apartment to see how she was doing. When she opened the door I could see from the look on her face that something was wrong. Before we could even sit down, a detailed description of her frustration tumbled out.

She had entered the hospital over a week before with a terrible feeling of pressure in her chest and extremely high blood pressure readings. While she was there, the residents caring for her had ordered numerous tests, but no one had told her the cause of the problem. Carlotta recognized a prescription they gave her as a medication that had given her a rash the year before. Although her infectious disease (ID) clinic doctor had pulled her off this prescription once already, she was forced to argue fiercely to be switched to another one. Most importantly, she was never allowed to talk to the supervising physician overseeing her care: "No one knew enough to tell me what the problem was. Finally, one student told me, 'I think . . . I assume, that it was an inflammation of the stomach [causing your symptoms]' I *think?* I *assume?* And what does the stomach have to do with the chest?"

In the end, Carlotta returned home confused and angry. She was already scheduled for a follow-up appointment. "I'm going to have to argue with them to get my questions answered," she told me in Spanish. "I don't like to argue, because I don't want my blood pressure to go up. But I see that I'm going to have to do it!"

This wasn't the first time she had encountered problems. On another occasion, her doctor referred her to an endocrinology clinic. Here, too, she was examined by residents who left to consult with their supervising physician and later returned with a prescription. But Carlotta understood that only the supervising doctor could approve her treatment plan, and she wanted to ask him directly about possible side effects. She also wanted to know exactly what was wrong but had not been able to get a clear picture from the residents who examined her.

When Carlotta asked to speak to "el doctor grande" (the head doctor), she was told that her prescription was all she needed and she shouldn't worry about it anymore. Determined to get more information, she persisted. She wanted the doctor to answer her questions about the medication he had prescribed and she wanted to know exactly what was wrong with her. "I don't like being disagreeable—*pero me dan pastilles y no explicaciones* [but they give me pills, not explanations]!

Like many others who worked with me, Carlotta felt that residents should never treat patients by themselves. "The head doctor should take students around with him, so they can watch him ask questions and take notes. But, to not even bring the head doctor along?" She told me that despite her protests, she was never allowed to talk to the doctor who wrote her prescription.

Experiences like these were very common for women like Carlotta, who were experts in their native cultural capital but uncomfortable with the *habitus* of white middle-class professionals, much less the culture of biomedicine. These women were usually uncomfortable in large hospitals and clinics. A few preferred Spanish to English, although not all did. But they all experienced discomfort with most of the professionals responsible for their care. When women like Carlotta attempted to advocate for themselves, they were often overruled or overlooked by clinic staff and health care professionals. Faced with the frequent repetitions of this pattern, they often adopted avoidance strategies, minimizing their interaction with hospital physicians and larger clinics. After months or even years of frustration, they began skipping monthly clinic appointments, either missing their checkups entirely or substituting visits with small Latino agency-based clinics whenever possible.

Women like Julia and Deborah, who were comfortable with the *habitus* of middle-class professionals, used the health care system differently. They explored the range of hospitals and clinics available and found professionals who could refer them where they wanted to go. Once they had chosen a clinic or hospital, they cultivated relationships of trust with at least one key physician, and usually with several. In this way, they built broader social-capital toolkits by creating networks of powerful allies. These women influenced their doctors, therapists, and social workers to make sure they got the best treatments available. They carefully managed the impressions they made on doctors and staff in order to achieve this end. Often, they worked hard to distance themselves from any suggestion of addiction or promiscuity. And though they could not avoid the stigma of AIDS completely, they deemphasized any parts of their history that included drug use or sex work. Michele Berger's study of HIV-positive women in

Detroit explored the power of intersectional stigma in the lives of her study participants. The multiple stigmas with which they grappled made them particularly vulnerable to ill-treatment at the hands of the clinicians and social service workers they depended on (Berger 2004). It is this kind of stigma that the women I worked with sought to avoid.

While women with broad cultural capital became successful self-advocates, women with average capital found themselves overwhelmed. Battered by each failed attempt to be heard, they lost confidence over time. This had profound consequences for their health and well-being, and it limited the benefits they could extract from a health care system dominated by a white, middle-class *habitus*. However, women with average capital reported better experiences in small neighborhood clinics, preferring doctors who shared their *habitus*. But since most HIV care was provided by infectious disease clinics in larger "safety net" hospitals that provided care to the uninsured and Medicaid patients, they found themselves outside their comfort zone again and again.

Welcome to the Clinic

Most of the women I worked with had Medicaid if they had insurance at all. Recall that Medicaid is the nation's medical insurance program for those living below the poverty level. As U.S. citizens, the women in my study could apply for Medicaid if they had no other coverage. If their incomes were low enough, they might qualify for Medicaid. But qualification was far from certain. Women in my study whose husbands worked were often turned down (as in the case of Luchita and Paquita), even though their spouse's wages were too low to pay for any kind of insurance coverage, if employers even offered it.

Finding a local private doctor who took Medicaid wasn't easy in Newark, and even fewer of these specialized in HIV care. This is a pattern common to poor, urban communities of color (Abraham 1993). However, safety-net hospitals and federally qualified health centers that provide care to underserved populations do take Medicaid. Many have infectious disease (ID) clinics specializing in HIV care. I found that facilities like these dominated women's experiences of professional biomedicine. They returned to their ID clinics again and again, and the relationships they developed with clinicians and support staff there impacted the length and quality of their lives more than any other kind of professional medical care.

Field notes from the summer of 1997 describe the Marshall ID clinic. A single rotating fan cooled the long, hot waiting room. It was packed with at least forty-five people at any given time. The two unisex bathrooms were accessible only through the receptionist. There was no easy access to food. Vending machines were ten minutes, and several floors, away. The sugary junk they dispensed was the only option for people who forgot their own snacks. Chairs were plastic, unpadded, and uncomfortable. One public phone sat in the center of a waiting room wall. The atmosphere combined shopworn dinginess with institutional gloom. Posters in Spanish and English bombarded patients with thinly veiled health propaganda from pharmaceutical companies and the Department of Health. In all the hours I spent there, I was the only person who took reading material (like *Poz* magazine and educational pamphlets) from the drooping literature rack, and I only did so out of a desperate desire to escape. To make matters worse, one of the receptionists (who was fired during the course of my study) and one of the nurses (who was not) were infamous for being disrespectful and just plain mean.

The long waits were disturbing for other reasons as well. A steady stream of people filed in and sat down over the course of three hours, and everyone in the room had ample time to examine them. For many, this meant coming face-to-face with people and possibilities they would rather not see at all.

For women raising young children, it meant watching a parade of HIV-positive children wander in and out of the room on family support days. As mothers, they reacted with pain at the sight (or thought) of HIV-positive children. Flor worried about transmitting the virus to her unborn child. Others remembered the terror they had faced waiting for their children's test results. Some wondered who would take care of their children after they were gone. Deborah put it this way: "I never go on Wednesdays. That's when the babies are there. I look at them and want to cry."

Excessively thin patients provoked universal anxiety when they arrived in the waiting room. Protease inhibitors had made AIDS-related wasting less common than in the past, but no visitor could avoid skinny, sickly patients forever. The women I accompanied wondered if they were looking at their own future as frail patients hobbled by or were wheeled in by relatives and friends. The first time Nini took me to the clinic she pointed out an emaciated man and said, "Welcome to hell."

A noticeable number of people in the waiting room looked totally impoverished. They arrived in worn, ill-fitting, or haphazardly assembled clothes. Some were clearly ill while others were vacant-eyed. My companions whispered that they were addicts, prostitutes, or just plain dangerous.

"Exactly why is the waiting room a problem?" I asked Carlotta. She explained that, except for early morning appointments, waiting rooms were full of "bad people. . . . [Only] the people who go to their appointments early are regular workers." Carlotta told me that the thinnest "look like drug users"; she thought that most of the women had probably been prostitutes. Others in my study thought so too. Nilsa confessed that the clinic waiting room always made her want to go home. "They [the uninfected world] already think I must be a prostitute or a drug user because of this [HIV]. I don't want to be here. I don't belong here." Despite their discomfort, the women I worked with were typically trapped in the waiting room for several hours at least once a month.

Women who used the clinic had little or no continuity of care. Even when women scheduled appointments around "their" doctors' availability, last-minute changes were common. Despite this, they persisted in trying to develop a strong relationship with "their" doctor. Broader social capital conveyed strategies for managing this problem:

> By the time Alicia arrives, there are many people in the waiting room. She is annoyed because she very specifically made an appointment with Dr. B and she got a call yesterday saying he wasn't going to be here. Dr. V was available, but Alicia put her foot down. She hates Dr. V. She would have canceled her appointment and waited had she been forced to see him. "The secretary knows I hate Dr. V and won't see him, so she got me an appointment with Dr. P," she said. (Field note excerpt 1999)

Most patients had files thick with the twists and turns of repeated opportunistic infections and complicated drug regimens. No doctor could review them, conduct an exam, and prescribe the best treatment in the ten or twelve minutes available. Only continuity of care could ensure good results. Because of this, women were leery of physicians who barely knew them.

NINI: Did you see that guy with the beady eyes, the one that looks crazy?

SABRINA: The one with the white hair?

NINI: I saw him once. He's a terrible doctor. He didn't know anything. If Dr. Sergio's gone, I leave. He's the only one that knows me.

LUCHITA: Sometimes the clinic is OK, sometimes it's not, because you see different doctors. It's supposed to be confidential then you have these students coming in that you don't even know, and this is the first time you're meeting them.

Women with average cultural capital and women stigmatized by drug use or sex work were at a major disadvantage during consultations. Those with histories of addiction fared the worst, but frustrated women who voiced their resentment (like Nilsa) were also given short shrift. It didn't matter that they were angry about the challenges they faced and the resources they lacked. Weary, overworked doctors simply couldn't invest in everyone who came looking for help, and they tended to avoid patients who seemed problematic. Doctors were more likely to invest their time and expertise in women with whom they were comfortable. They were less likely to invest in women they found threatening, alien, or unfamiliar. Shared cultural capital translated into fifteen minutes of consultation time (as in the case of Nini and Dr. Sergio) instead of six (as in the case of Carlotta and Dr. Vincent, which will be explored shortly). But women with average cultural capital often had so little in common with the doctors who treated them that they could not establish this kind of rapport.

As was the case in Berger's study, clinic physicians were wary of patients they suspected of drug use or sex work (Berger 2004). Doctors told me they anticipated being lied to by substance users looking for prescriptions to sell on the street. This was a potential problem: one day Nini took me to see groups of men selling medications and painkillers on the black market not far from the clinic. In all fairness, medication sale was a legitimate concern for ID clinic doctors. But it was impossible to know for certain which patients would take their prescriptions and which ones would sell them. Nevertheless, patients suspected of drug use had a more difficult time getting prescriptions of all kinds, and it was especially hard for those in recovery to get painkillers. I saw both Nerina and Cristina ask for pain medication that was refused.

Appointments were always short, but they were noticeably shorter for those suspected of addiction, those with a history of sex work, the severely depressed, and patients who were angry. This often meant that those most in need tumbled to the bottom of the pile and had to make due with whatever they could extract from an unsympathetic environment. My observations showed that they often received "assembly line" care. Carlotta described a monthly clinic appointment for women with average cultural capital:

> The only thing he says is "How are you? How's your appetite? Are you vomiting or experiencing diarrhea?" Then he comes over, looks me over and says, "Open your mouth—breathe—" and that's it! [He says,] "Are you out of any medications? You have all of them? You don't need anything?"

Carlotta went on to tell me that when she was out of medications, she told her doctor and he simply said, "OK, OK," and gave her the prescription, ending the encounter. When I actually began observing her monthly consultations with Dr. Vincent (a pseudonym, as are all names used here), he asked exactly these questions in precisely the order and manner she described. And when I glanced at my watch as we walked out of the room together, I realized that her appointment had taken a total of six minutes.

Although Carlotta experienced the briefest consultations I witnessed (followed by Paquita), repeated observations established that ten to fifteen minutes was all the time most clinic patients were given. Unless residents were being trained, only a few moments were allotted to the communication of complex, potentially life-threatening problems. Those who took too long were cut off so the standard routine could be initiated. A few of the clinic doctors I observed made an effort to speak with their patients in a more focused, extensive way, but this was not the norm.

I noticed that nurses placed more emphasis on communication; they usually obtained more complete descriptions of the day's problem. Residents were also more likely to solicit narratives and listen while women explained their symptoms. In these cases, women faced the opposite problem: they grew tired of repeating themselves to an endless succession of people. When residents were involved, I found myself prompting weary women as they told their stories to a nurse, a resident, and finally to the supervising doctor. By the last round, they were so tired that they sometimes omitted critical information.

Nadia and Nini Visit the Clinic

Nadia was a slender woman with a boyish haircut when I met her. Nini pointed her out to me, saying she was an active drug user. I insisted Nini introduce us in the clinic waiting room. I told Nadia about my project and asked if she would like to be part of it. She agreed and invited me to tag along during her upcoming consultation.

We talked for about an hour while we waited. Nadia impressed me as a shy, retiring person. During that time she explained that she was in recovery from drug use, describing her struggle to maintain sobriety. She lived with a boyfriend who used and sold drugs. He constantly pressured her to take them. She told me she had refused most of the time, but had given in on several occasions. Now she was afraid she would have to leave him to stay away from drugs. The emotional distress of ending their relationship was complicated by the fact that he was paying the majority of the rent and leaving him meant trying to find (and finance) another place to live. In a city where safe, affordable housing was extremely scarce, this was a real challenge.

On top of everything else, her new HIV medication regimen had produced serious side effects. She had taken them once, but the side effects had been so distressing that she stopped after her initial attempt. She hoped her doctor would switch her to another set of medications that day. As our conversation progressed, Nadia made it clear that her life was packed with challenges and her stress level was very high.

When she was called back to the consultation room, she reiterated her invitation, asking me to accompany her. Interestingly, the physician she saw that day was Dr. Sergio, Nini's trusted and beloved doctor, whom I had observed caring for Nini many times before. Once inside the consultation room, Nadia sat on the examination table and told Dr. Sergio that she had stopped taking her new HIV drugs because they had provoked intense anxiety and severe disorientation. She searched his face for a response as she described her disoriented responses with animated gestures. But Dr. Sergio turned his back on her almost as soon as she started talking. She continued to plead her case to his back while he examined her file, refusing to make eye contact. After a short silence, Nadia asked why she hadn't been able to recognize her own face in the mirror after she had taken the new prescription. Why had she felt so anxious? Why had she been confused?

But Dr. Sergio did not answer. Nadia asked him to change her medications and write her a different prescription this time. He remained silent. With hardly a word, he scribbled out some prescriptions and handed them to her. Nadia and I walked out of the room together looking at the scripts. They were prescriptions for exactly the same combination of drugs that had elicited her side effects. Nadia stared at them and did not say much. She left the clinic rather quickly.

Almost immediately afterward, I went back into the consultation room with Nini for her monthly clinic appointment. From the moment she walked in, the two of them began smiling and laughing like old friends. Dr. Sergio listened to everything Nini said with great care and attention. He maintained constant eye contact. He examined her body carefully, checking for thrush in her mouth and asking her about any problems she might be having. He never hesitated to touch her. His affection and respect were so obvious that I found it hard to believe that he was the same man I had watched turn his back on Nadia only fifteen minutes before.

As I returned to the clinic again and again over the following months, I looked for Nadia. I asked other patients about her, but no one could tell me they had seen her. One fall afternoon, I walked into the waiting room and sat down, only to hear someone calling my name. I looked up to see a gaunt person yelling in my direction. Peering closely, I couldn't tell whether the baggy shirt and secondhand hat concealed a man or a woman. But I nodded hello as the caller rose from a chair and began hobbling toward me. The person repeated my name, asking, "Do you remember me?" With shock, I realized I was looking at Nadia, now twenty pounds lighter and half crippled. My shock and horror must have shown on my face, because as soon as I hugged her she began to cry.

She told me that this was her first time back in the clinic since the day we had met. She was very sick and had been living on the streets for months. Her boyfriend had used the rent money to buy drugs and they had been locked out of their apartment. Then he had abandoned her. At first she had slept in the hallway but the landlord had threatened her so she left. Her daughter, tired of dealing with an addict, had refused to take Nadia in.

Nadia had been in pain for months; every time she urinated it hurt. Her entire abdomen hurt. She had no place to sleep, bathe, or go to the bathroom. She did not have the money to eat regularly. Her voice trembled as she tried to explain it all. I put my arms around her and stroked her head. "Since you have been so sick, why didn't you come back?" I asked quietly. "Because Dr. Sergio treated me so badly the last time. I cried and cried after I left," she said, weeping. "I was so ashamed. You were there. Don't you remember?" "I remember," I answered sadly.

Referrals and Test-Result Roulette

When ID clinic doctors encountered problems they could not manage, they referred women to other specialty clinics, usually part of the same health system. Often they were located only a few floors away. But files, records, and test results regularly disappeared en route from one part of the hospital to another.

> Celestina walked to the front area reception desk to check in. As she stood and waited, the receptionist was looking for something. "Well it's either here or in . . .," I heard her say as she rushed off. Celestina wandered back and rolled her eyes. "They lost my medical record," she told me. "It's happened to Roberto a few times. I always check to make sure they have my medical records. I'm never relaxed until I see that they have them. See, they are seeing other people first because they can't find my records." (Field note excerpt 1998)

Patients with broad cultural capital sometimes obtained copies of their test results and hand-carried them to future appointments, but not all clinic personnel allowed patients access to their records. Yet busy nurses could be convinced to make photocopies of important test results for patients with the right kind of cultural capital.

I observed numerous cases in which important test results did not make it to a clinic by the first or even second successive appointment, a delay of two to three months. Consider such a delay in the context of Newark's early HIV epidemic: when researchers first began tracking survival rates, women lived for fewer than four months past their initial diagnosis (Leusner 1990a)! Even today, when ID clinic doctors refer patients out for the tests that inform challenging treatment decisions, obtaining timely results can become a problem. Such test-result roulette hinders continuity of care by blocking communication between clinicians (as in the case of Flor's OB/GYN and ID teams, discussed in chapter 2).

Average Capital: Avoidance and Substitution

Women with average capital responded to these obstacles by avoiding them. They either minimized the time they spent in the clinic (by booking early morning appointments or choosing doctors who moved quickly) or they skipped regular appointments unless they were ill or needed something. Monthly appointments could sometimes be replaced by three-month check-ins if a physician thought a woman was doing well. For women with average capital, and some in the middle, this could be a huge relief.

> When I feel in the mood to go I go make my own. . . . They give me the appointment but I never really go when they give me the appointment. I make my own appointment. I go whenever I want to go. I go just how to see my T-cell is and, you know, when to get ready to take my blood work? Like it's really, I mean that's every three months. So why go to the hospital every month, why to? Just to see my face? I ain't got time for that, you know. *Amelia*

To tell you the truth, I like [this clinic] better. I think it's just they treat you faster and, you know, I hate to go to doctors, to the hospital, so I want to go to somewhere that's fast and quick and get it over with and take me home, you know? That's it. Give me what I need and that's it. *Nilsa*

Sometimes women could get blood pressure monitoring or preventative care at small agency clinics. When it was possible to substitute agency visits for ID clinic visits, women with average capital would usually do so. In general, though, women with average capital had more difficulty keeping all of their (many) appointments. Flor had both ID clinic and OB/GYN appointments. Nilsa and Paquita had ID and neurology clinic appointments. It is important to acknowledge, however, that these symptoms and side effects made it difficult to pursue the treatments that would relieve them. If women woke up feeling ill and exhausted, it was easier to stay in bed than maneuver the city in a crowded bus for ten minutes' audience in a crowded clinic.

Broad Capital: Improved Access and Better Care

Most hospital admissions occurred through the ER, although in some cases, women were hospitalized for scheduled cancer treatments or diagnostic tests. The women I worked with usually preferred one hospital over others. But those with average capital rarely had the opportunity to select the hospitals to which they were admitted. Women of broad cultural capital, however, maneuvered their referring physicians or therapists skillfully to ensure placement at the facilities of their choice. These women assessed the strengths and weaknesses of each local institution and decided where to go in advance of each admission, depending on the condition for which they would be treated. Nini, for example, chose one hospital for a cancer operation but another for a two-week stay in the mental health unit. She collaborated with her doctors and therapists to arrange admittance into the facility she preferred for these very different conditions.

Women of broad cultural capital also had more agency in deciding where to obtain HIV care. Some, like Nini, followed their favorite physicians to an ID clinic and invoked strategies like calling ahead and building rapport to circumvent the poor conditions they encountered there. Others uncovered alternatives to safety-net ID clinics. Two of the "high capital" women I worked with, Nerina and Julia, consulted Dr. Hamilton, a physician who used several small consultation rooms at Mercy Hospital to maintain his own practice. It was located half a building away from the Marshall ID clinic, and he was one of the very few local nonclinic physicians who both accepted Medicaid and had extensive experience with HIV-positive patients. Nerina and Julia had initially both used the Marshall clinic, but they disliked it so much (as did most clinic users) that they had switched to Dr. Hamilton's practice instead.

When I first discovered this I asked them how they had found Dr. Hamilton. I knew that the Marshall clinic saw Medicaid clients, but I had assumed that "private" doctors—including nonclinic, hospital-based HIV specialists—would not accept Medicaid patients. But both Julia and Nerina (who had Medicaid) assured me that Dr. Hamilton accepted Medicaid and that he was available to the same patients who were now using the clinic. "But why aren't all those other unsatisfied clinic users seeing Dr. Hamilton as well?" I asked. Nerina only shrugged, but Julia said, "They probably don't even know about him."

Field notes from my first three visits to Dr. Hamilton's practice describe the striking differences between the two environments. Clinic patients often waited hours to be seen. Dr. Hamilton's patients chatted with each other for twenty to forty minutes before being seen. I saw no more than seven or eight patients in the small, carpeted waiting area during peak hours. Across the hall from the waiting room was a clean, wheelchair-accessible bathroom.

The group assembled in Dr. Hamilton's waiting area looked as if they had just left a high-rise office or might return there after they left. Although most of his patients were either African American or Hispanic, I saw a greater proportion of white patients than I had seen in the clinic. Everyone dressed, spoke, and presented themselves as educated, financially stable, white-collar workers. Finally, most of the patients I encountered in his waiting area looked vigorous and healthy. Although I saw one or two slender people, I encountered no emaciated patients.

Later, both Julia and Nerina told me that this environment was an important reason that they switched from the clinic to Dr. Hamilton's practice. Both explained that they hated the waiting room at the clinic because of the unsavory people there, the ugly waiting room, and the long waits.

> Oh God. It was terrible [at the clinic]. People wanting to buy drugs. They don't care, they just go there for the drugs. And now that when they're in trouble, they be crying, ya know? Then they want help, and it's too late. I guess [the doctors at the clinic] give 'em their stuff [medications], and they come back and say they lost it, they were ripped off and so they treat everybody the same way, as if they're junkies. I wasn't going to be subjected to that. So that's why I moved to Dr. Hamilton, you know, on a one-to-one basis.

Unlike ID clinic patients, Dr. Hamilton's patients could see him every time they visited his office. As his patients, they had continuity of care. Observing his consultations, I noticed that Dr. Hamilton remembered both Julia and Nerina every time he met with them. He readily recalled details of their treatment history and past conditions. Without looking at their charts, he could begin conversations about the outcomes of previous medication changes or recent trends in viral load. Consultations occasionally ran over the fifteen-minute mark, and they were much more personal, unlike the highly routine consultations I saw in most ID clinics. Dr. Hamilton's process varied according to each patient's condition and concerns, and his solid relationships with Nerina and Julia meant that he remembered details of what happened in their lives as well as their bodies. Many of the clinic patients I observed could not even begin to expect these things. In short, from my perspective, Dr. Hamilton offered them higher quality care.

Dr. Hamilton's patients also benefited from all the services that ID clinic patients received and more. He could arrange specialty referrals more easily than clinic physicians, and if his patients were admitted to the ER, he was usually advised of the problem quickly. Recall his ability to intervene when Nerina broke her foot and needed a cast, as described in chapter 2. This did not always happen quickly enough; Julia told me that she was once in the hospital for two days before Dr. Hamilton was consulted. But even this was better than many clinic patients could expect; his close relationship with his patients meant he was more useful to them when they were in the hospital.

I noticed that Dr. Hamilton monitored his patients' use of supplements, herbs, and home remedies, supporting them in their use of these CAM modalities. I once saw him suggest that Julia add milk thistle to her daily vitamin regimen to enhance her liver's functioning. I observed that he considered exercise and balanced diets so important that he took the time to ask about them. When I compared the care Dr. Hamilton gave Nerina and Julia with that of most of the average-capital clinic patients in my study, I realized that Nerina and Julia received more attentive, more comprehensive care.

> I got Dr. Hamilton, and if I'm down, you know he knows, I mean he would refer me, and if there's an OB/GYN problem, he's on top of things . . . but when you go to clinics in the hospital, it's a monthly, bimonthly checkup. Do you understand? And it's just, a big caseload, they see so many people and they don't have the time. I walk in with a lot of people a lot of times to accompany them, and the doctor is already like, "What you need?" [said quickly and harshly]. Do you understand? A lot of times they don't even look at your throat or listen to your chest, they don't do that! In this clinic it's like the patients are over there and the doctor is over here, you know, it's like a barrier in between. *Julia*

And though security guards at the hospital told me that Dr. Hamilton's patients were assumed by hospital personnel to have AIDS, I noticed that his patients were stigmatized less often by hospital staff than ID clinic patients.

However, not all clinic patients received poorer quality care. Women with broad cultural capital and those in the middle sometimes formed strong relationships with clinic physicians, as in the case of Nini. I observed that these women were more likely to receive consistently attentive, more personalized care, and their relationships were warmer and more affectionate than those of their average-capital counterparts. A direct field note excerpt from 1999 describes this kind of doctor-patient relationship.

> Alicia and I are waiting for only a moment when Dr. Bach comes in. He is much older than I expected: in his fifties, at least. He wears a tweed coat— he's a very handsome and distinguished older man. He has white hair and a short, well-groomed white beard and mustache. When he speaks, it is clear that he is European. He has piercing blue eyes that examine a person very, very closely—they look right into you.
>
> He greets Alicia with gruff affection. She is so happy to see him! She is bubbling with happiness. He sits down, no white coat, no nothing. He looks at the file, but mostly, he looks at her. She is talking to him about her pelvic pain and he alternately looks at her and then at the file—He is obviously listening to her, or doing an excellent job of faking it.
>
> She introduces me and I explain a little of what I am doing. He looks at me very directly, then says to her: "She will publish all your secrets if you're not careful." Alicia smiles and tells him no, not to worry. But he persists in looking at her. I say, "I will show what I write to Alicia and if she says not to publish something, I won't." He seems to be measuring me. He is protecting her—or trying to protect her—from me. I am glad to see his tenderness for her, although it feels a little uncomfortable.
>
> As he looks at her file, he says, "Do you know that Dr. Raymond had you tested for drugs?" with a kind of contempt in his voice. She is really surprised. No, she exclaims—he says yes, he ordered a drug test for her. She is angry and upset and she says so. Dr. Bach is also grimly angry. Alicia goes on about how she *never* does drugs and never has. But how could he think that she was taking drugs? Dr. B. goes on—"He also administered a pregnancy test"—he is chuckling in an annoyed way, as if at the stupidity of this. Alicia is also floored. She tells us that she is not sexually active and hasn't been for over a year. She could *not* be pregnant.
>
> Dr. Bach looks at me and says, "They don't listen to their patients. They don't believe them; I do." It is a simple, powerful statement. It resonates in my head. He continues to affirm that most doctors don't have the courage to *ask* their patients and listen to them. He does. His attitude is simple. Dr. Raymond did some stupid things. His manner, his not-listening, is stupid. Alicia clearly agrees with this.
>
> Now Dr. Bach asks her about her pain and how it has been manifesting. She still has pain in the pelvic area and lower back. But it's not usually the case any more that she feels pain urinating, or that she feels a need to urinate but can only squeeze a few drops out. He listens. He tells her that the results of the tests that he sent her for last week are normal,

too. When she asks, he carefully goes over the medications that she is taking. He remembers most of them without asking her. He takes a moment to tell her that one of the medications that she is taking can cause very small particles of gravel, not big enough to show as stones. . . . As we walk out of the building, I am struck by the intimacy and collaborative nature of their relationship.

Recent primary care research has focused on the healing dimensions of intimate doctor-patient relationships. A qualitative study of "exemplar healers" and their long-term patients has described three key physician processes that foster healing relationships: creating a nonjudgmental emotional bond, consciously managing clinician power in ways that benefit patients, and displaying a commitment to their care over time (Scott et al. 2008; Scott et al., 2009). While I was not able to observe the women I worked with long enough to establish a history of long-term commitment, repeated observations allowed me to observe examples of nonjudgmental bonds and consciously managed clinician power in the most intimate doctor-patient encounters, as exemplified by Alicia's encounter with Dr. Bach. I was also able to see the enthusiasm that women in these kinds of relationships expressed for their physicians.

Broad Capital: Building Social Networks and Treatment Plans

Although women with broad cultural capital and some women in the middle began as supplicants at local clinics and hospitals, they did not stay in this role for long. They quickly developed relationships of trust with key personnel who worked there. In clinics and hospitals, they sought out doctors and nurses who habitually invested in their patients and developed rapport with them. Sometimes they did so by reflecting the *habitus* of each potential ally back to them and speaking, moving and acting in ways that were comfortable and familiar to the person to whom they were talking. Pierre Bourdieu calls this kind of concrete physical performance *embodied cultural capital* (1983).

> After we sat down [in the waiting room], Nini jumped up to talk to A. and S. [clinic nurses]. I stood next to her feeling uncomfortable. . . . All three began comparing their elaborate nails and chatting gaily in Spanish about their last manicure while they laughed and waved their hands around. I tried to hide my chewed-off nails, but A. saw me and smiled surreptitiously. It reminded me how long it's been since I got my hair cut. I felt kind of ugly and wanted to sit down again. . . . Dr. Sergio greeted Nini and they began to talk, [and] her voice got softer. Her Spanish shifted, too, becoming more formal. She didn't talk with her hands like she did with the nurses, but she kept eye contact and so did he. [Field note excerpt 1998]

In some cases, women did this in a calculating way, but most of the time they unconsciously deployed a nuanced, genial affect that fit right into the cultural context at hand. Embodied cultural capital helped women work the system, or more accurately, "systems," since the health care organizations they used were made up of smaller, interlocking organizations, each with its own unspoken rules. Women who used embodied cultural capital well quickly learned which kinds of behavior resulted in longer, more personalized consultations and which ones didn't. They also worked hard to subsume those parts of their history that were most likely to threaten or alienate doctors and medical personnel.

For example, Nini made sure that everyone who worked in the clinic knew that her husband had given her the virus. She emphasized that she had been legally married to a middle-class man with a secret past. By publicly referring to what her husband had done, she established herself as an innocent victim who didn't "deserve" HIV. This doesn't mean she faked her anger; it just means that she understood its ability to solidify her reputation as a respectable woman. It was no accident that broad-capital women could inspire empathy quickly and easily. Their canny use of impression management and embodied cultural capital was a crucial relationship-building skill.

Emerging Patterns

All the women in my study disliked sitting in ID clinic waiting rooms. They hated it not just because of the long waits and poor conditions, but because these environments forced them to face terrifying possibilities (a wasting death, transmitting HIV to their children) and stigmatizing identities they rejected (addict or former addict; prostitute or ex-prostitute).

In response, women developed a variety of strategies for avoiding the clinic waiting room. Those with average capital and some in the middle made early

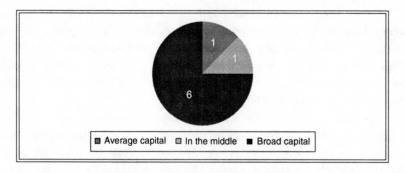

FIGURE 6.1 Strong Clinician Alliances

morning appointments and/or deliberately chose doctors who gave fast, cursory care (like Carlotta and Luchita). Some skipped regular clinic appointments whenever possible (like Nilsa and Amelia), and most substituted visits to local agency mini-clinics when the opportunity arose. Women with broad capital and some women in the middle either found alternative private physicians (like Nerina and Julia) or built close, healing relationships with clinic physicians (like Alicia and Nini).

Women with broad capital expended tremendous effort to establish a strong rapport with one key physician. Whether they attended a clinic or saw a private physician who accepted Medicaid, they worked hard to encourage their doctor to take a personal interest in their care. Cultivating physicians was important because continuity of care was important, and intimacy facilitated longer, more personalized encounters and better care. Impression management and embodied cultural capital were used to solidify these doctor-patient relationships.

Women with average capital were less likely to believe it was possible to establish a strong, caring relationship with a doctor. Some made multiple attempts to establish relationships and get more personal care, as in Carlotta's case. Others had already given up by the time we met and just tried to avoid their medical appointments as much as possible, as in Amelia'a case. Of the eight women who successfully established strong clinician alliances, only one was a woman with average capital; another fell in the middle. Most average-capital women made due with the limited relationship and cursory care they already had.

Women with broad capital were more likely to work collaboratively with their doctors in multiple ways. They asked for, and got, a significant say in their care. Recall Gabrielle's chapter 2 comments about her relationship with her doctor: "a little bit of them and a little bit of mine makes it perfect," and Nini's ability to prompt her psychiatrist for a helpful mental health diagnosis. Alicia was also able to ask for, and receive, a comprehensive review of all her medications. Even more critically, she obtained her doctor's trust, and the actions he took in designing her care were framed by that trust (remember, unlike Dr. Raymond, Dr. Bach never attempted to test her for drugs or pregnancy against her will).

In other words, women with broad capital worked well with physicians who were willing to engage in collaborative partnerships. In this regard, they were like "expert patients," who learn as much as they can about every aspect of their illness and actively contribute to the design and delivery of their care (Lorig 2002). Unsurprisingly, these women were more likely to see their doctors when they felt sick instead of avoiding them.

It is important to remember that broad-capital women were unusual. Their ability to adapt to the *habitus* of key people in their lives was extraordinary. Most people, including many of us reading this book, can't just step outside of our native *habitus* whenever it's convenient for us to do so. But that is exactly what broad-capital women did. None were raised in white, middle-class families, but previous exposure had enabled them to adapt as needed. It is this flexibility that is extraordinary, not their facility with white, middle-class culture in and of itself. Women with average capital were like the majority of us: comfortable in our own neighborhoods, businesses, and institutions, and nervous when forced to step outside of them. Most of the time, their lack of flexibility wasn't a problem; it was just a normal behavior that became a serious disadvantage in hospitals and clinics.

I did witness several women (Nini, Julia, Nerina, Celestina, and Caridad) try to help friends and acquaintances acquire this flexibility. These attempts usually faltered. It was too much to ask women with average capital to absorb a lifetime of experience in a few months, and unreasonable to try to distill the insights of a broad toolkit into a simple list of clinic "dos and don'ts." Cultural capital takes time and ongoing exposure to build, and women without extensive, ongoing support or a preexisting foundation on which to build could not catch up to their more successful peers quickly.

But the fact remains: average women and men should not have to suffer simply because they struggle to step outside of their day-to-day worlds. Our health care system should not reserve consistently good care for only the most extraordinary among us. It should be equally responsive to everyone. The excellent care enjoyed by Newark's most flexible women underscored the cursory care received by the rest. In Newark's urban health care system, you had to be exceptional to get good care.

7

Taking Care of Yourself

> I feel tired when I go out and, you know, all I wanna be is in the house. I'm not like before that I used to be running here and running there, and you know, now it's like, I wanna be comfortable, you know, in the house, in my house. Not in nobody's house. Not like before I used to do, like to get up and get dressed and open the door and go out and go shopping, and go walking here and walking there. Now, no more. So then when I'm back I'm a mess. My feet hurt, my body is all aching. *Alicia*

For Alicia and her cohort, HIV meant an increase in the demands of daily living. Families still had to be cared for; households still had to be run; and, as noted previously, women often supported HIV-positive husbands or partners as well as their children. In addition to these obligations, women now had to make time for ID clinic appointments, specialty care appointments, support group meetings or mental health care appointments, and a daily regimen of pills and remedies.

Making sense of these demands was overwhelming. Each woman found herself sifting through them, trying to determine what was necessary, what was worth exploring, and what was untenable. The way in which each woman approached her postdiagnosis life was directly related to the range of cultural and social capital on which she could draw.

Women with average cultural capital were more likely to conserve their energy whenever possible. They cut back on what they expected themselves to do, reduced travel, and prioritized rest. Often, their low energy levels made it even harder to take advantage of resources and allies. This group of women sometimes preferred to focus on home remedies over clinic visits, as in the case of Carlotta and Luchita. Their participation level was lower than that of their counterparts with broader cultural capital; they were more likely to complain of chronic symptoms and side effects. Women with average capital were also more likely than their peers to drop treatments—even helpful ones—because the energy required to maintain them proved overwhelming.

Women with broad cultural-capital toolkits did not follow this pattern. They rarely complained of low energy levels. Instead of slowing down, they added new projects to their lives: investigating a wide range of home-based treatments, exploring new CAM therapies, and looking for previously over-looked strategies to improve their health. And because they aggressively sought out anything they thought could help them, they occasionally pushed themselves to the point of exhaustion; these women were more likely to experience periodic acute episodes requiring hospitalization.

Women with broad capital were more likely to continue using their chosen treatments until either the benefits diminished or a better approach was found. They were less likely to drop treatments that helped them because of low energy levels. Finally, they were more likely to adhere to home-based and CAM treatment plans consistently over time than were women with average capital, but they refused to slow down and rest.

Compelled to Rest

I almost always try to lie down, to lie down and be comfortable. Or sitting comfortably, but preferably lying down. *Carlotta*

Bed rest, or extended periods of inactivity, was very important to women with average capital. They often told me that resting could strengthen the immune system and reduce both the frequency and the acuteness of symptoms. Increased sleep was credited with rejuvenating powers, as was staying home for long periods. This was believed to cut down on emotional and physical stress and gradually build up strength, although several women acknowledged that it could also be a sign of depression. Those who reported frequent, wrenching fatigue tended to downplay or ignore the latter view, however. Alicia, who landed somewhere between those with average capital and those with broader capital, also held these beliefs.

Women with broader capital strenuously rejected the power of bed rest. They believed in lingering at home only when symptoms were acute. They said they felt best when interacting with others, usually through socializing, volunteering, or working. They usually argued that isolation made them feel worse, not better. I sometimes witnessed arguments between women in this group and their partners or older children about the wisdom of resting at home. Nini described one such argument it this way: "I had another argument with Justicio [her boyfriend], a big one. He says I have too many friends and I am never in the house resting during the day. I say, 'Well, if there is nothing to do there, why stay?' But I do have too many friends. And he says that I need to take care of myself. I never take care of myself. He's right about that." In these exchanges, family members attempted to push women into sleeping later, staying in, and recovering their strength. I never saw this argument succeed. Although bed rest was used by every woman I worked with during periods of serious debilitation, it was the method of last resort for women with broader capital.

Low Energy: Alicia, Cristina, and Amelia

Shortly after we met, Alicia described the lifestyle change she experienced after her diagnosis. In her old life, she had thought nothing of leaving home everyday to do chores, visit friends, and pursue the outside world. But once she began treatment for HIV, simple local travel became too exhausting. The day after a trip, her body ached and she felt irritable, sometimes for several days. For her, managing chronic illness meant a kind of self-imposed isolation.

Of course, this kind of shift would have been nearly impossible without substantial help from family and friends. On some days, she couldn't even manage with their help—particularly in regard to childcare. As the mother of three children, Alicia's caregiving responsibilities could be lessened, but they could not be eliminated.

> Sometimes, most of the time [I have to] force myself to do the things around the house, because my body is still aching. . . . more than half of the time my body is aching. I don't feel like getting up and doing this, but if I don't do it, who is gonna do it? So I have to force myself to get up and clean the house, do the laundry, and necessary tasks.

When she had to do housework, Alicia pushed her body to do the minimum work required and asked her children to help: "See, I told my son, 'You clean tonight' [and he said] 'OK mom.'" Because Alicia's husband had died several years before, she depended on her children to help her manage the tasks of daily living. Her mother often shopped for her, and other relatives and friends stopped by to do small chores, or they brought food and helped with laundry. She was fortunate to have an unusually large family living close by and lucky to have willing children, old enough to help. After HIV/AIDS activist Nelson connected her with other women like herself, she was sometimes able to draw on their assistance as well. Selma often visited her and eventually moved next door. Because of this expanded social network, Alicia was able to work less and rest, while conserving precious energy. But not all the women I worked with were so fortunate.

As an isolated single mother, Cristina found herself managing her health while caring for a teenage son, her brother, and a new boyfriend. Recall that because she had moved to New Jersey from another state in the past six months, she had no local family. Only the three men in her household could assist her, and most of the time they didn't. This threatened her health and made her deeply unhappy. It added stress to the challenges she already faced as an impoverished HIV-positive woman of color. And though she recognized that she would benefit from a lifestyle shift that lessened her responsibilities, she couldn't make the change without help. She described the situation this way:

> Like right now, my brother lives with me, and my son, and my boyfriend, you know, he stays here all the time. And you know there's times when I'm sick and those dishes go without washing, you know, and . . . the house will be a mess, a wreck, because they won't do anything, you know? And then so that makes it hard for me. 'Cause whenever I do get up outta bed [chuckles], I have to start cleaning and doing everything around here . . . and I wonder what they would ever do if I wasn't here. Because you know, my son is fourteen, he's old enough, to do things, and he doesn't, you know. . . . I should be tougher on that but . . . sometimes I just get so sick that I just want to lay down and I don't want to hear it, you know . . . so if I had to tell 'em to do something I usually end up arguing about it.

Though Cristina realized she could press her household for help, she didn't think it would work. She expected her family to argue about it, worsening her stress levels. As difficult as it was to meet her household's demands while ill, she thought it was better than fighting with her family and then doing the work anyway. To cope, she tried to do everything possible when she felt good and then lie low when she felt bad, coping as best she could by herself.

Her resignation also reflected the impact of internalized and external gender roles on the lives of the women with whom I worked. These roles were a significant factor in Cristina's household drama. As Puerto Rican men, her son, brother, and boyfriend did not expect cleaning and cooking to be part of their daily lives (Massara 1989). Because of gender-role socialization, both Cristina and the men in her family assumed she would complete her "normal" household tasks despite periods of acute illness. If Cristina had lived with a daughter instead of son, her situation might have been different; a daughter would probably have been socialized to help her. If her female relatives had lived close by, she might have been able to ask them for help.

Like other women with average capital, Cristina believed in the rejuvenating powers of bed rest. She thought that if she could somehow slow down and drop some responsibilities, her immune system would be stronger and her quality of life would improve. Because of this belief, she tried to snatch rest whenever she could, despite the constraints of her gender role. But there were times when she felt conflicted about this, fearing that she was shortchanging her son. "I think he so, so relies on me, and, and everything because I'm the one that knows how to [do] the grocery shopping, pay the bills, you know, clean the house, cook the food . . ." She was not the only one to feel this way.

Many women told me that when they were extremely tired and they had no help, they were forced to drop essential tasks even though the consequences could be serious. This caused intense distress, particularly in mothers of young children. As Amelia confided in me with great shame, "You know, when I'm on this treatment [referring to fatigue-inducing HIV drugs], I don't, I don't wanna take care of them [referring to her children]. Because it, it hurts me. You know what I'm saying? And I have my son taking care of himself and his sister. 'Cause there's times when I cannot even take care of me."

Amelia explained that she believed she should take her HIV drugs because her doctor had convinced her that they could keep her T-cell count high and her viral load low. He had pointed to improved results after she started the medications. But in order to adhere to this regimen, she had to practice extensive bed rest as the drugs caused fatigue. This kept her from staying alert to the needs of her children, but the prospect of being immobilized and indifferent while her son and daughter played unsupervised filled her with alarm. In the end, she stopped taking the drugs altogether, even though she thought they could help her stay healthy, partly out of fear for the well-being of her family.

Women of average capital with young children were in the worst possible position. Although they wanted bed rest, they shunned it so they could take good care of their families. With little social support and no one to take over their most critical responsibilities, they felt they had no choice. In every single case, when one of the women I worked with had to choose between caring for her family and safeguarding her health, she chose her family over herself. This was true even when she believed the decision might hasten her death.

"I'm Just Lazy"

Six women with average capital told me they had dropped a home-based treatment that had significantly improved their health. Several said they were sacrificing their long-term good for a short-term benefit and weren't proud of it. Whenever they discussed their inability to adhere to practices or regimens that had helped them, they used language implying shame or embarrassment. "I'm just lazy," was a comment I heard again and again. "I'm too tired," was the less judgmental version.

Yet when I counted their daily responsibilities (household management, caregiving, crisis management, and sometimes income generation) or thought about their low energy levels, this seemed harsh. And when I added up the number of children and adults they cared for and considered the challenges of urban poverty, I could not agree that they were lazy. But I could see that they were often exhausted, ill, overwhelmed, and relatively isolated. I wondered how they were able to function at all. It was not difficult to understand why medical, home-based, and CAM treatments alike fell victim to the combination of low energy and average capital.

Carlotta's experience with juicing provides one such example, drawn from field notes. She discovered the practice through a Spanish-language radio program that suggested it might ease her symptoms. She decided to give it a try. Carlotta began by juicing several times a week. She praised it and told me that the juice relieved swelling in her legs and feet. This was important, since her swollen legs sometimes made it difficult for her to leave the house. She even had a walker for hobbling around her tiny apartment during an attack. Over time, the amount of energy required to buy the vegetables, make the juice in small batches, disassemble the juicer, wash it, and reassemble it became too onerous. At first, Carlotta tried to "stretch" her energy by making larger batches that could be refrigerated over two days. But she soon found that after just one day the juice separated and tasted foul. So she stopped. Sometime later, the swelling returned. Carlotta believed that her decision to stop juicing contributed significantly to her subsequent decline in health.

> I used natural juices because I had heard on the radio that it's good for people with arthritis to drink potato juice, so I drank it, but then I stopped. And I felt good, and I think that's what happened to me. While I was drinking the natural juices, I felt strong and good. I stopped drinking them and everything collapsed . . . when I stopped drinking them I began to get worse again, I became weak, I began to feel weak, and I said, well, I guess what happened was I drank that [the juices] and I was strong and then I stopped drinking them and I began to feel bad.

Although it created cognitive dissonance, women with average capital consistently made choices that required the smallest expenditure of energy possible, even if they believed a different choice would yield better long-term results. I found that an energetically demanding option that yielded an excellent outcome would be dropped in favor of a low-energy option with mediocre outcome. This was much less common among women with broader social capital.

Vitamins, Herbs, and Dietary Supplements

Many of the women I worked with explored the natural health movement, although women with broader capital pursued them with greater energy. The natural health movement refers to an eclectic system of self-care that utilizes a wide range of health practices and emphasizes the importance of disease prevention; it is often popularized through self-help books and health food stores. Through word of mouth or informal research, women became interested in vitamins, herbs, and the use of dietary supplements. This often meant taking high-dose vitamins (both alone and in combinations) and using herbs to target specific problems or functions like enhancing the immune system.

Herbs were often used in the form of teas. Ten women (most with broader capital) reported using them. These women intermingled elements of a Puerto Rican or Latino healing tradition with what they learned from the natural health movement. Quite a few women mentioned that herbal teas like chamomile, dandelion root, and parsley were used by family members to treat a range of conditions; some even asked their relatives to bring teas and dried herbs with them when they visited from Puerto Rico. Nini had received special training in the traditional use of herbs from a Cuban religious and herbal specialist, and she periodically used this knowledge to help herself and others.

> They taught me how to use it. A Palero [Afro-Cuban spiritual practioner] taught me, which is one of the most powerful people there are among the Cubans. He showed me how to prepare teas, how to deal with herbs for baths, and my grandmother taught me a great deal as well, 'cause I'm good at it, OK? *Nini*

Most women, however, did not use the full range of herbs that their parents and grandparents had used on a regular basis. They drew a few traditional herbs into their repertoire and expanded their knowledge through the natural health movement. But almost all of those who learned about herbs from a natural health perspective had been comfortable with the concept from the beginning because they had been familiar with the use of herbs in a traditional ethnomedical context. "Ethnomedicine" is a term that refers to health care traditions, beliefs, and practices of specific cultural groups (Singer and Baer 2007).

Costs mounted very quickly for those who used vitamins and herbs in capsule form. Multiple doses were often taken each day, and a bottle of thirty capsules ran out quickly. Supplements were expensive, with a single bottle costing between six dollars and twenty-five dollars, depending on the product. Other kinds of supplements, such as aloe vera juice (extracted from the leaves of the aloe vera plant) could also be expensive.

The high cost of supplements was a challenge. Money was tight for everyone, and most women depended on disability checks, welfare, or minimum-wage jobs (theirs or someone else's) to make ends meet. There was rarely enough to pay all the bills without sacrifice, much less buy luxuries like vitamins. In this context, every purchase had to be carefully weighed.

At one point, Celestina told me she felt guilty about drinking aloe vera juice because it cost so much. Most of the women who took vitamins and supplements expressed similar concerns. None of the women had access to lower-cost food cooperatives; they all shopped at health food stores, the most expensive outlets for natural health products. Cost was clearly a barrier to full participation, and everyone who used supplements said they wished they could take more of them. But women found ways to buy some of what they wanted the most, despite cost. Those like Nerina, who feared the side effects of pharmaceutical drugs, were especially committed to supplements.

As previously noted, most women had heard about a vitamin or herb's ability to resolve some health problem with which they struggled. Among the supplements they tried were aloe vera juice, molasses, cat's claw, shark cartilage, ginseng, and a range of vitamins. Women also tended to follow specific diets in conjunction with supplements; Nerina was a vegetarian and Carlotta ate a low-salt diet. Luchita had just changed her diet when she told me about her discovery of vitamins and supplements through a group of gay male friends:

LUCHITA: I'm just taking vitamins, eating beans, not greasy stuff you know . . . I do everything natural . . . we just have to watch what we put in our bodies because oh my God! . . . I know people that's taking it and they felt, hoo [face lights up and eyes brighten]!

SABRINA: Yeah? Who's doing that?

LUCHITA: I, like, three guys from [an HIV agency]. And they say they feel much better! I think it's better . . . the doctors say I'm crazy but . . . [shrugs]

Luchita explained that a small group of men attending a local support group had begun researching the natural health movement. They had started to explore some complementary and alternative medicine (CAM) instructional material produced by earlier groups of white gay men living along the East and West coasts. These materials (in the form of newsletters, magazines, and product lists for HIV/AIDS-related buyer's clubs such as those mentioned by Jeff Bomser, chapter 3) had encouraged the group to start exploring the utility of a wide array of vitamins and supplements. Although their project was frowned upon by local agency staff, the group persisted. Luchita knew these men through the local AIDS community and had just started consulting them for self-treatment advice. Like Nerina and Celestina, she was highly motivated to pursue these therapies because she experienced severe side effects from her HIV medications. She hoped to shift away from her drug regimen and move towards a regimen of herbs and vitamins.

> I always tell my husband ain't no virus gonna kill me, you know, it's these poison medicines they use. They all have side effects, [on] your kidneys, your liver, your pranca [pancreas] . . . some make your sugar go up 'cause that happened to me already. They took me off one because my suga' was shoof! Super high. I'm gonna get more into natural herbs and stuff like that . . . I'm gonna try to find out what's going on, cause this is a lot of people that's taking natural herbs. *Luchita*

Puerto Rican Women and Gay White Men: Divergent Understandings of CAM

Luchita was following in the footsteps of an earlier health movement when she turned to the local men's support group for treatment advice. Multiple researchers have documented the way in which affluent white men with HIV disease used alternative therapies in an attempt to redefine their circumstances, consciously taking control of their own health management rather than relinquishing it to their doctors (Whittaker 1991; Anderson et al. 1993; Furin

1995). These men became what Kate Lorig calls "expert patients," or patients who "take responsibility for day-to-day decisions about their health, and who work with health care professionals as collaborators and partners to produce the best possible health given the resources at hand" (Lorig 2002, 814).

Jennifer Furin's 1995 dissertation, "Becoming My Own Doctor: Gay Men, AIDS, and Alternative Therapy Use in West Hollywood, California," describes how the men she interviewed tapped into their considerable cultural capital (my term, not hers) to become expert patients, integrating CAM therapies into their medical treatment plans. She explains how they learned to interpret their own test results and conduct literature reviews on drugs, herbs, and dietary supplements (Furin 1995, 116, 288). Her work demonstrates how these men used their education and social privilege to infiltrate the medical world, appropriating the tools and specialized information they found there for their own ends. Many used their expertise to help create a large network of grassroots organizations designed to teach HIV-positive people across the country about CAM therapies of potential value. The pioneering advocacy work of middle- and upper-class gay men was described in more detail in chapter 3.

There are enormous differences between the affluent white men who pioneered CAM's use in HIV disease and the marginalized Puerto Rican women of Newark. The clearest differences lie in the tremendous gap in cultural and social capital between the two groups: none of the women that I worked with could draw on the *habitus*, education, or elevated social status of these men. Even women with broader cultural capital did not command this kind of privilege. However, there is another difference as well: for these pioneering gay men, CAM was situated outside of any familiar cultural context. In fact, many forms of CAM, such as acupuncture, were drawn from cultural systems that were completely foreign to them. Crossing outside of their *habitus* and reaching for forms of medicine alien to the West was an act of resistance to the political, cultural, and medical systems that were allowing HIV-positive men of that period to die.

But the women I worked with all had some familiarity with the use of herbs to treat illness. And all had grown up surrounded by Santeria (a Caribbean religious tradition combining African and Catholic belief systems that includes a range of medicinal and spiritual healing practices) even if they did not practice it themselves. None had been indoctrinated with the body-mind split that characterizes professional Western medicine. Even women with little or no previous interest in the ethnomedical traditions of their families knew about them and had seen them in use. Many may have adopted some parts of the worldview (s) that underpinned these traditions. For the women with whom I worked, the use of ethnomedicine and parallel practices from the natural health movement was more like coming home than rejecting home.

Even those who repudiated some part of their ethnomedical tradition (like Santeria) held onto beliefs (about the power of prayer, for example) to promote healing that derives from it. Rather than using alien practices to claim their right to health management, the women I worked with embraced older patterns of self-care, looking for easy ways to manage their symptoms and side effects. Not surprisingly, this generated a very different understanding of CAM than that of white, middle-class gay men.

Non-ethnomedical CAM in Newark

It was easy for Newark's resourceful women to turn to Santeria or herbalism; Newark is home to many ethnomedical practitioners. For those opposed to such practices, charismatic Christians offered spiritual healing. But it was more difficult for women to find other forms of CAM. Because of Newark's economic and political history, their choices were much more limited than would have been the case in cities like New York and San Francisco. Unlike those cities, Newark did not have an affluent, white gay community when HIV arrived. As noted in chapter 3, most of Newark's gay community was poor; its members had little of the middle-class cultural capital required to bring CAM to their aid. IV drug users and their families were at a particular disadvantage. New Jersey's affluent PWAs spent the early years of the epidemic looking for CAM in New York City, leaving Newark's poor behind (Hancock 2002).

However, recall that Bill Orr, a former member of ACT UP, and colleague Jeffery Bomser helped import some of New York's affluent cultural and social capital when they worked to establish the North Jersey Community Research Initiative (NJCRI) in 1988 (Whitlow 1988b). The AIDS Mastery Workshop, run by Northern Lights Alternatives, was another transplant. It was offered in the Newark area as early as 1992. This two-day workshop used acting techniques to help empower HIV-positive people and their loved ones to meet the challenges of AIDS (Patterson 1993). The workshop was taught by New York-based actors with the support of other AIDS activists. Its privately funded volunteers were a good example of the kinds of collectives that brought CAM to Newark. Despite organizations like this, however, Newark's limited resource base failed to attract a wide range of CAM practitioners.

Many of the women I worked with wanted to try non-ethnomedical forms of CAM. To do this, they depended on initiatives funded by the Ryan White Care Act, NJCRI, or agency-sponsored workshops as described in chapter 5. Acupuncture was especially popular; free, ongoing local treatments were made available to HIV-positive residents of Newark and Elizabeth as part of an ongoing clinical trial. Acupuncture may also have been attractive because of its use in the treatment of drug addiction; I frequently encountered individuals in recovery from addiction using it to reduce drug cravings.

Massage therapy was also available at no cost through a social service agency, although it was not as popular. The therapist who provided it worked outside of the immediate Newark area and few of the women I worked with owned cars. Julia described it like this:

> Pero nena [but honey] it's so far away! They [the massages] are not accessible for us . . . and the acupuncture—forget it! You have to go to Montclair, not Newark. You're gonna tell me to hop on a train and spend half an hour on the bus? You gotta take a day off! You've got to leave your house in the morning and travel and travel . . .

Some were also reluctant to use this service because the therapist was male. Still, acupuncture and massage therapy were the most consistently funded and readily available forms of non-ethnomedical CAM available to those with whom I worked.

Most women wanted a personal, ongoing relationship with a CAM practitioner who oversaw their care. They would have preferred to avoid using social service agencies as intermediaries. But without the Ryan White funding that made these services free, none of them could have afforded it. They were dependent on social service agencies that used Ryan White funding to hire CAM practitioners. As Luchita explained, "I would like to find a natural doctor like I don't have no insurance no nothing. I can't go to a natural doctor. How they gonna get paid?" The funding that made CAM available also governed the length of its availability. Alicia, Luchita, Caridad, and Nini all stopped using non-ethnomedical CAM when their Ryan White–funded practitioners moved too far away. Luchita and Nerina tried to replace them with local practitioners that they could afford with mixed success. And Julia, Gabrielle, Luchita, Juana, and Carlotta each told me they wanted to use some form of CAM more frequently, but that without Ryan White's funded services, they couldn't afford it, even if they could find it.

Some agencies sponsored CAM workshops or sent clients to conferences that offered them. Women with broad capital had strong relationships with agency staff, which allowed them to take advantage of these opportunities. One summer the Union County HIV Consortium sponsored a women's support group focused on CAM therapies; it brought in speakers and practitioners, and women who were part of that agency's network were able to participate. Agencies also provided transportation so women could attend the annual NJWAN Women and HIV Conference, where massage therapists offered free massages to HIV-positive women in a dedicated hotel suite.

Self-Care Strategies for Depression and Anxiety

Every woman I worked with experienced bouts of sadness, depression, or anxiety, with only one exception, Luchita. Not surprisingly, they all had strategies with which to manage them. Some would be familiar to almost anyone: Deborah favored long, hot baths to promote relaxation, for example. But many were highly individualized. Women with broad cultural and social capital reported the widest range of strategies to combat depression and anxiety. Women with average capital were much more likely to explain that they stayed home and slept for long periods whenever they felt depressed, as in the case of Juana, Amelia, Cristina, and Nilsa. Women with broader capital, however, reported a wide range of creative and unusual strategies for managing sadness and stress.

Celestina fought chronic anxiety for at least a year while her doctors pushed her to start combination therapy, also known as HAART (highly active anti-retroviral therapy), which consists of three different kinds of drugs to be taken together in a strict sequence. Doses can't be missed for fear that the virus will mutate and become drug resistant. Adhering to this extraordinarily regimented kind of treatment is difficult, and those who try often struggle with it. Most difficult are the side effects: vomiting, nausea, headaches, extreme fatigue, vivid unpleasant dreams, body aches, and changes in body fat distribution have all been reported (Correll et al. 1998; Moore 1999; Ives, Gazzard, and Eastbrook 2001; Arici et al. 2001; Maisels, Steinberg, and Tobias 2001).

Initially, Celestina rejected the recommendation. She had watched her husband, Roberto, experience new side effects every time he switched combinations. At the start of each regimen he vomited continuously and was generally miserable. In addition, some of the drugs caused liver damage or diabetes (HHS 2005). Celestina knew all about these problems, having seen Roberto meet challenge after challenge in hopes of keeping his viral load down.

She did not want to deal with any of these side effects and had experienced none of the opportunistic infections that made treatment seem urgent. But as her T-cell levels eased down and her viral load crept up, she became depressed. When her doctors told her to start treatment or prepare for serious illness, Celestina believed them. She accepted the idea that she needed combination therapy to stay healthy. Yet watching Roberto, she could not bring herself to begin taking the drugs.

DR. PATEL: You need to be on HIV medication. Your T-cells are dropping. They are at twenty now.

CELESTINA: I was on medications for awhile but they made me vomit. It's in my head now; I don't like to think about taking them.

DR. PATEL: I don't want to pressure you . . . there will never be any pressure, but I want you to come in next week ready to start medications. Do whatever you need to do to be ready.

Celestina is silent and looks down at her hands Later, she tells me miserably, "It is my decision, but my T-cells are so low I should take them. Nothing can help me except the medications. But I don't want to think about this anymore!" [Field note excerpt 1999]

Field notes covering a span of several months tell the story of this period. As Celestina got more miserable, Roberto started to worry about his wife's long-term health, so he teamed up with her doctors to pressure her into taking HIV-treatment drugs. Celestina responded by getting intense migraine headaches. She stopped sleeping at night. The situation was further complicated when she reluctantly started a drug regimen but had to quit on the third day because of severe nausea. During this period, she met with a psychologist every week and entered a stress-management study for HIV-positive women, but the backbone of her plan to stay sane centered on solving jigsaw puzzles.

When her children were at school or she couldn't sleep, Celestina put together dozens of puzzles. At first she allowed no one else to touch them, and as she finished, she covered each one with contact paper and framed it, hanging it on the wall of her apartment. After a while she let her sons join in, but she always did the majority of the work herself. Assembling puzzles helped her manage the ambivalence she felt so pressured to resolve. Of course, while this drama unfolded, Celestina was scrambling every day to meet the laundry list of requirements laid down by welfare, HOPWA, and SSDI. She told me she would have gone mad without puzzles. For her, puzzles were the best form of mental health care.

Gabrielle had a similar experience. Her memory was becoming spotty and her long-distance marriage caused her stress. As noted previously, she spent most days caring for her small granddaughter and dealing with an adult son who showed no inclination to support himself. HIV landed low on her list of priorities, but demanded attention nonetheless. Whenever she got overwhelmed, she painted. She didn't paint landscapes or portraits: she painted and repainted the walls of her apartment. "People ask me why my apartment has different colors, when they come in and see [my place] . . . when I feel upset I like to paint, to paint a wall, and then I feel relaxed, Mami. When I was in jail I painted the whole church."

She showed me all the different colors of all the different walls and pointed out areas where work was still in progress. As soon as she started to feel bad, she chose a wall and began covering it with another color. When she felt better, she stopped, leaving the wall partially painted. She had changed the colors of her walls many, many times. It made her feel better when she was especially depressed.

Reaching for Divine Assistance

For many of the women I worked with, spiritual support was as important as material support. Religious beliefs provided hope in difficult times. Women's spiritual practices were remarkably diverse. Luchita and Nilsa belonged to Pentecostal churches. Carlotta practiced a blend of Catholicism and New Age beliefs; Nerina and Julia blended New Age with Santeria. Gabrielle and Nini focused only on Santeria, and Juana was a Jehovah's Witness. Celestina, Caridad, and Deborah were Catholic, but Caridad was thinking of joining a Pentacostal church. Selma, Alicia, Amelia, Cristina, Flor, and Paquita rarely spoke of religion and did not appear to be religiously observant. The range of practices, beliefs, and strategies in this small group of HIV-positive Puerto Rican women was exceptional. (See Loue and Sajatovic 2006 for more about the spiritual support among urban Puerto Rican women.)

Both Pentecostal women and the sole Jehovah's Witness invited church friends to lay hands on them in times of stress. New Age women created rituals to restore their mental and emotional balance.

> My pastor lays hands on me, yeah, and anoints me with oil like the word of God says: "Those who are sick, anoint them with oil, the holy oil and pray over them for healing." She's done this for me a lot of times in church. And then you feel good 'cause you feel like a peace coming over you, you know, that's what the word of God says. And to anoint your house with oil, too. *Luchita*

> I also try to energize my chakras [referring to her body's energy centers] and I do everything that I possibly can do that's within my reach. Because when I keep all my energy within myself, that's what is going to prevent, that will always keep me well. *Carlotta*

Practitioners of Santeria kept small, unobtrusive altars in their homes. They also used spiritual techniques to resolve depression, ill health, and bad luck. Catholics sometimes maintained home altars as well, lighting candles to the Virgin during hard times. Sometimes these categories proved arbitrary; I saw Deborah, a Catholic woman, mixing creative visualization with the lighting of a candle to the Virgin Mary.

Nini Banishes Depression

One day Nini decided that she was under so much stress that her health was starting to suffer. She explained that although she was seeing a therapist, her sessions were not enough to bring her relief. She needed a bath, she said. "A bath?" I asked, perplexed. Delighted at my confusion, Nini instructed me to look out her bedroom door. Mystified, I watched while she dashed down the stairs to the chain-link fence that separated her yard from her neighbor's. I saw her stick her fingers through a gap in the fence, grab a tall weed and pull it toward her. She quickly snapped off a piece and tucked it into her pocket.

Turning around, Nini glanced up at me and smiled broadly. I waited for her return even more puzzled than before. When she walked back into the kitchen, I asked what she had been doing. Laughing, she explained that she was stealing a bit of "ruda" from her neighbor, who had a nice big plant. She said she always took some of that ruda when she needed to give herself a bath. Reaching into her pocket, she produced a sprig of herb I would later identify as rue. After letting me sniff it, she filled a glass with water and plopped the little green stem inside.

Then Nini told me exactly how she was going to use it. Later in the week, she would take me to a special store where she could buy a small bottle of patchouli oil. Then she would put the sprig of rue in a clear glass container with some sugar and patchouli and cover the whole thing with water. She would let it sit overnight and then use the rue to sprinkle the liquid over her head and body after her shower. This would clear away all the bad influences around her and help her feel better.

When I asked where she had learned this, Nini told me that her grandmother did it in Puerto Rico. "My grandmother thought it worked against evil spirits. But, no, I don't believe that. It takes away depression and stress." Nini didn't dismiss the concept of "spirits" completely, but she believed in the bath's rejuvenating powers rather than its literal ability to banish evil spirits.

This description was taken from a single field note written in 1999, but I saw Nini recommend baths like these on multiple occasions. She was careful, though, to hide her use of Santeria and herbs from Pentecostal friends like Nilsa. This didn't always work, since statues of the Orishas (deities or spirits honored by practioners of Santeria) were visible to those who peeked into her bedroom. Sometimes Nini argued with Nilsa, who thought Santeria was evil. Occasionally, Nini expressed conflict about the way her spiritual practices angered her Pentecostal friends. Eventually, though, she began associating less and less with these women, choosing the traditions of her youth over her relationships with them.

Nini did not restrict her use of Santeria to the direct treatment of ill health. She used it to solve all kinds of serious problems. Recall that when she appealed SSDI's rejection of her second application, she decided to consult a Santera (a religious specialist in the practice of Santeria). She also found a legal aide and solicited letters of support, but this matter was so important that all possible strategies had to be invoked. The Santera decided that a special ritual was needed to ensure that the judge who heard Nini's disability case would decide in her favor. The two women went to a poultry farm, selected a chicken for sacrifice at the ceremony, and enacted the ritual before her final disability hearing. Between her letters, her legal aide, and the ritual, Nini was finally granted disability status.

Emerging Patterns

Almost all of the women I worked with experienced HIV-related symptoms, medication side effects, or both. Women with average capital were more likely to report chronic symptoms or side effects, and women with broad capital were more

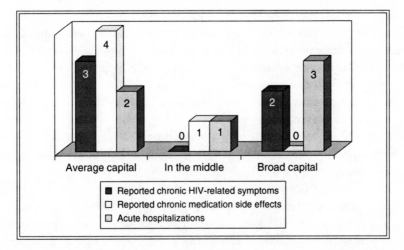

FIGURE 7.1 Symptoms, Side Effects, and Acute Hospitalizations by Cultural-Capital Category

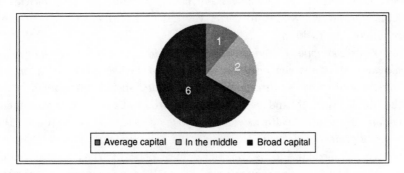

FIGURE 7.2 Strong Support Group Alliances

likely to report periodic acute hospitalizations. Women in the middle fell somewhere in between. It is possible that chronic illness hampered women's ability to generate social capital. It is also possible that average social capital indirectly aggravated chronic illness. It seems likely these patterns coexisted. Women with broad capital were much more likely to push themselves to the point of exhaustion and become seriously ill, even when their families urged them to exert themselves less.

All the women I worked with faced overwhelming demands, but the two groups met them in different ways. Women with average capital conserved their energy, cut back on their responsibilities, and depended on family members for help. Those without family to assist them and those with small children suffered the most, skimping on self-care to provide for the people they loved. These women tended to themselves with whatever energy they had left over. As a whole, they had smaller support groups and social networks than women with broad capital. Broad-capital women, however, reached out to their large social networks for the support, assistance, and therapies they needed. They used their allies to help them take care of both their families and themselves. These women spent much more time and energy looking for resources and building connections than their counterparts with average capital. Of the nine women with strong support group alliances of various kinds, only one was a woman of average capital.

Both groups of women were interested in complementary and alternative therapies, but women with broad capital tried more of them. I noticed that women with broad capital pursued *all kinds* of therapy more vigorously, more frequently, and more successfully than women with average capital. Neither group expressed a preference for either medical treatment or CAM for reasons of ideology or political resistance. But women with average capital did prefer home remedies and home-based CAM over clinic visits, while women with broad capital spent more time and energy pursuing both medical experts and CAM providers. Neither group was willing to travel very far or dedicate an overwhelming amount of time to do so.

With the exception of Nerina and perhaps Luchita, none of the women I worked with saw CAM as a form of resistance to the hegemony of biomedicine or the stigma projected on them by mainstream and medical culture. In fact, the women in my study did not see CAM and biomedicine as antithetical. Only Nerina, who spent years in the natural health movement, spoke of CAM as a way to contest the power of professional medicine; she was the only one who believed CAM and professional medicine to be in philosophical opposition. As my study progressed and Luchita began talking with a local HIV support group for gay men, she began to express similar sentiments. But this shift in Luchita's attitude, if underway, was very much in process during my study.

Exposure to their own ethnomedical traditions led the women I worked with to interpret unfamiliar forms of CAM as variations on healing practices they already knew. This primed them to see CAM as a way of relieving symptoms and side effects, not as a pathway to agency or political empowerment. In this way, their experience of CAM differed from that of the white gay men who popularized its use in the early years of the U.S. HIV/AIDS epidemic (Whittaker 1991; Furin 1995). However, it did parallel the experiences of HIV-positive people around the developed world.

Many studies have showed remarkable agreement regarding CAM use among the HIV-positive. They found an extremely high use of alternative therapies concurrent with the use of HAART and other pharmaceuticals. Estimates of CAM utilization rates among HIV-positive individuals range from 67 percent to

84 percent (Sparber et al. 2000; Knippels and Weiss 2001; Standish et al. 2001; Gore-Felton et al. 2003). This trend holds true throughout the industrial world; European studies confirm the findings (Agnoletto et al. 2003). Commonly used therapies include nutritional supplements, herbal medicines, marijuana, massage, acupuncture, meditation, imagery, yoga, and aerobic exercise (Fairfield et al. 1998; Greene et al. 1999; Duggan et al. 2001; Standish et al. 2001; Gore-Felton et al. 2003).

Studies found that CAM use among HIV-positive individuals was intended to address drug side effects, improve energy levels and fatigue, combat stress and depression, and improve quality of life (Calabrese et al. 1998; Fairfield et al. 1998; Patrick 2000; Pawluch, Cain, and Gillett 2001; Thorne et al. 2002; Wu et al. 2002). Few users completely abandoned biomedicine in favor of CAM, although this was occasionally observed (Thorne et al. 2002).

In one study, women were shown to be four times more likely than men to use CAM than men, and they used more, different kinds of CAM at the same time than did their male counterparts (Gore-Felton et al. 2003). In another study of African American and white HIV-positive women, 60 percent used at least one form of CAM. With the exception of acupuncture, the most common therapies reported mirrored those preferred by Newark's resourceful women: vitamins, religious healing, herbs, dietary supplements, and massage (Mikhail et al. 2004). It appears that the help-seeking strategies of Newark's resourceful women were not so unusual after all.

8

Learning from Resourceful Women

I began my work with Newark's resourceful women by asking four key questions. Given their limited resources, how did they manage an illness as serious as HIV/AIDS? Did they seek out alternatives to conventional medicine and, if so, what kind? Could they act as effective agents despite the structural violence that constrained them? And what could Newark's resourceful women teach us about our health care system and the way we can expect to use it?

How Did they Manage HIV/AIDS?

The key differences between more successful and less successful women can best be understood through Pierre Bourdieu's concepts of cultural capital, *habitus*, and social capital. Remember, cultural capital refers to the class-specific knowledge, values, preferences, and skills that dominate the social environment, or *habitus*, in which individuals are raised. Social capital refers to the body of potential resources that can emerge from relationships of trust. Though all of the women I worked with were raised in a marginal- or working-class Puerto Rican *habitus*, some had also been exposed to other ways of seeing and knowing the world, through education, institutionalization, and recovery programs.

These women absorbed some of the cultural capital of groups other than their own. A few could even draw on the embodied cultural capital (body language and speech patterns) of those other groups. No matter where they were or who they were with, these women were able to appear relaxed, gracious, and culturally competent. They made their acquaintances feel at home, so they built

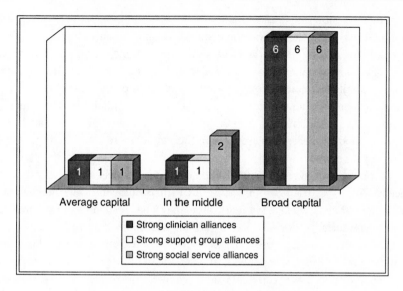

FIGURE 8.1 Ability to Form Strong Alliances

alliances with ease (see figure 8.1). People of all backgrounds wanted to help them, so they got better advice, better support, and better care than other, less flexible women who actually needed it more. In Bourdieu's terms, these women's diverse cultural capital enabled them to build greater social capital, which in turn enhanced their well-being and perhaps, in some cases, lengthened their lives.

Women with average cultural capital were like most of the rest of us: comfortable and relaxed in our own *habitus*, but tense and confused outside of it. In their own neighborhoods and local organizations, these women understood the unwritten rules guiding interpersonal behavior and could interact with other people easily. Outside of familiar settings, they didn't know what to expect or how to operate, so they struggled, sometimes even alienating those who could help them. This kept them from building the social capital that could have vastly improved their lives.

In terms of illness management, women with broad cultural capital approached HIV/AIDS with the same strategies they used to manage their other problems. They canvassed local agencies, government bodies, safety-net hospitals, and federally funded clinics in order to understand what was locally available and who controlled access to each resource. They built dense networks of allies, turning to these allies whenever they needed help. Because they could cross from their own *habitus* into those of others with relative ease, their networks were socially and ethnically diverse. Many of their allies were middle-class professionals with direct access to the resources they needed, like expert medical care or admission into agency support programs. And though the help of these middle-class professionals was important, it wasn't the only kind of help they needed. For finding under-the-table work, for example, they turned to allies who knew how to scramble for unofficial jobs. Because women with broad capital cultivated all their connections carefully, they could count on the help of just the right person whenever a need arose. The social capital they accumulated through these relationships gave them access to the best clinicians, facilities, mentors, and social services available in their area. It also connected them to a range of street-smart friends.

Women with average capital worked harder to meet their basic health needs. They, too, tried to build alliances with people who could help them. Sometimes they succeeded, but more often, they failed. Watching them, I noticed how uncomfortable they were in environments dominated by middle-class professionals and those different from themselves. These women struggled to cross out of their own *habitus*. In general, they depended more on their relatives than did women with broad capital. Average-capital women also battled chronic fatigue, medication side effects, and HIV-related symptoms more than their broad-capital counterparts.

This study was not designed to clarify the relationship between chronic physical symptoms and social capital. Because of this, it is unclear whether chronic poor health was an outcome of average social capital, or whether it inhibited women from building it. This is a question for future research. However, it is clear that women with average capital were less likely than women with broad capital to persist in getting the kind of care they wanted. After months or years of trying and failing to work with alien bureaucracies, they often became discouraged, withdrawing even further into their own family circles.

It's important to note that women with broad capital also struggled with health challenges. Because they pursued so many avenues of care and support, they sometimes pushed themselves to the point of exhaustion. And though they reported less of a day-to-day struggle with chronic physical symptoms, they experienced more acute hospitalizations than their average-capital counterparts. Women with broad cultural capital typically refused to slow down, increasing the likelihood of adverse events. For them, illness management revolved around acute episodes rather than chronic symptoms and side effects. However, women with broad capital did not report feeling overwhelmed or physically devastated by the help-seeking process, as did their average-capital counterparts.

It's also crucial to remember that broad-capital women were not the norm. Their ability to adapt to the *habitus* of others was extraordinary. Most people can't simply step out of their native *habitus* whenever it's advantageous to do so. But broad-capital women did it on a regular basis. None were raised in a white, middle-class *habitus*, but when they encountered it in clinics, hospitals, and agencies, they could adapt as needed. It is this flexibility, this talent for social shape-shifting, that was extraordinary, not their mastery of white, middle-class cultural capital per se. Their successes emerged from their flexibility.

Broad-capital women had a distinct advantage when they tried to incorporate new health practices into their lives. Perhaps because they could count on plenty of help, they didn't constantly fight fatigue the way women with average capital did. And because they were more successful at self-advocacy, they tended to build collaborative, healing relationships with their doctors and health care professionals, working with them to co-create treatment plans they could live with.

Although women with average capital tried to adopt new health practices, fatigue and limited social support interfered with this process. Able neither to sustain healthy behaviors nor lean on others for support, they could not actualize their own agency or exert much power over their worlds. From this perspective, "agency" can be seen as a product of broad cultural and social capital. Women with broad capital were able to function as successful social agents in most circumstances, while those with average capital were not. This pattern persisted across multiple domains, manifesting in a variety of ways throughout women's lives. Pragmatically speaking, women with broad capital were much more successful at accessing economic resources and obtaining high quality care (see figure 8.2).

At least one important question remains: exactly what kinds of experiences led to the accumulation of broad capital, and what sort of life history characterized women without it? As I explored this question, I found that both groups of women included almost equal numbers of persons with English-fluency issues.

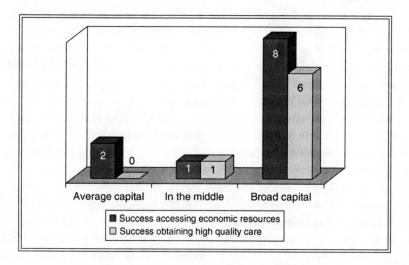

FIGURE 8.2 Success by Cultural-Capital Category

The average-capital group was dominated by island-born women, but the broad-capital group was split equally between the mainland and island born. Parenting did not appear to matter: every woman I worked with was a parent, and the majority had children at home. Living with others did not appear to be connected to average or broad capital, nor did the presence or absence of a husband or long-term partner. But broad-capital women reported more years of formal education, more exposure to institutionalization, and more participation in formal recovery programs than women with average capital. I argue that it was this broad exposure, either through education, incarceration, or recovery, that appeared to explain the difference.

How Do Newark's Resourceful Women Use CAM?

When it came to the use of complementary and alternative medicine or CAM, the women I worked with had a great deal in common with HIV-positive people living in other industrialized nations. Like them, they used a wide range of CAM therapies to improve their energy levels, reduce fatigue, and ease drug side effects. In this regard, their use of CAM offered no surprises, except, perhaps, in the sense that their poverty didn't stop them.

Their low incomes did not keep them from exploring CAM, because the therapies they used most often either required no out-of-pocket expenses, as in the case of Ryan White-subsidized acupuncture and massage, or they fell into the rough category of ethnomedicine: herbs and teas that were affordable and readily available. Prayer and spiritual healing were also common and usually free. Low incomes were most likely to keep women from using unsubsidized therapies and expensive supplements.

Unlike the white gay men who introduced CAM to AIDS care in the United States, the women I worked with did not see CAM as a political or ideological tool. Instead, they interpreted it through the lens of their own ethnomedical traditions. Rather than using foreign practices to assert their right to self-determination, Newark's resourceful women followed older patterns of self-care, looking for easy ways to manage their symptoms and side effects. Unfamiliar forms of CAM were associated with familiar ones: Reiki and energy healing were compared to Santeria or the Christian practice of laying-on of hands, and unfamiliar supplements were likened to herbal teas. Not surprisingly, this generated a very different understanding of CAM than that of white, gay men.

For Newark's resourceful women, CAM was an accessible way to respond to the demands of their illness. Unlike gay men, they did not see CAM and professional medicine as radically opposed. Instead, they saw both as healing tools for their bodies, minds, and spirits, all of which needed care. However, broad-capital women behaved more like their white, gay predecessors than women with average capital. Broad-capital women aggressively pursued CAM and

Western medical options alike. They negotiated with their doctors to get what they wanted and they advocated for themselves and others. This overlap between the broad-capital women I worked with and white, gay men who dominated the early epidemic can be attributed to both groups' relatively high reserves of cultural and social capital. Both had resources with which to demand attention from the health care system and both used it extensively, becoming like "expert patients," who could speak with authority about their illness, educate doctors when necessary, and shop for the best care available (Lorig 2002).

What Kind of Power Do Newark's Resourceful Women Have?

Social scientists have questioned the agency of impoverished urban women of color at risk of contracting HIV. They have pointed out that such women may have little or no power to control their risk, or to find treatments and resources once they have been infected. They urge us to refrain from over-representing women's power to determine the conditions of their lives. This caution is wise. But the problem is complex: how can we keep from overestimating women's agency without obscuring the power that they do possess? Based on my work with Newark's resourceful women, I suggest that cultural and social capital plays a critical role in facilitating or blocking impoverished women's agency.

Even in an environment plagued by poverty, violence, limited resources, and a crumbling infrastructure, Newark's broad-capital women can exercise their agency. They can significantly improve the quality of care they receive, even under highly unfavorable conditions, and can probably extend their lives as well. Social capital, built on a broad foundation of cultural capital, enables women to exercise their agency by drawing on the resources of their allies. But though women with average capital also try to exercise agency, they are rarely successful outside of familiar social settings. They can be effective social actors within their own *habitus*, but are more likely to stumble when they attempt to leave it.

However, the real question is not whether poor urban women can exercise their agency: it is *why* they must do so to get consistent, high-quality health care.

Listening to Resourceful Women

When discussing cultural and social capital, it is tempting to focus only on ethnicity. Research confirms that we face a wide range of racial and ethnic disparities in health and health care. National debates encourage us to focus on health issues related to race and national origin, and there are many excellent reasons to do so. The impact of disparities on the health and well-being of men and women of color is devastating. But cultural capital is class specific as well as (sub)culture specific, and once we acknowledge its role in facilitating or imped-ing access to high quality health care, we are forced to consider the impact of social class as well as race and ethnicity on the health of all marginalized and working-class people.

This study makes it clear that we must do a better job of creating structures that do not punish the chronically ill and those unfamiliar with institutional culture. Even people raised in a middle-class *habitus* are confounded by the norms and practices of hospitals, doctors, and clinics, but for the chronically ill (and urban HIV-positive in particular) it is much worse. They are placed in the untenable position of trying to weave together multiple sources of care and sup-port while running households and raising families. It is almost impossible to extract good care from the safety-net system under these conditions; only women and men with the highest reserves of cultural and social capital have any hope of doing so. As many have pointed out, the urban "safety net" is not designed for people who must manage a severe chronic illness and take care of families at the same time. Any real change in our health care system will have to tackle these problems by adopting a centralized, cooperative approach to health that promotes self-care alongside of family care.

Expanded, more accessible primary care may offer part of the answer. Recently, there has been a great deal of discussion about the next model for pri-mary care in the United States: the PCMH, or "patient-centered medical home." This refers to a new, as yet unrealized way of structuring family practice offices and clinics that allows them to provide more collaborative, team-based care (Crabtree et al. 2010; Rosenthal 2008). Innovations that help patients develop strong healing relationships with their health care professionals have the poten-tial to ease the burden of chronically ill people and their families. So does "inte-grated care" that facilitates easy access to a diverse range of specialists and health care practitioners within one institution (Boon et al. 2004). However, the PCMH and integrated care are probably only early steps in the transformation of our health care system (Crabtree et al. 2010). Deeper changes will be required to make sure that health care professionals have the time and support they need to care for patients with complex chronic illnesses. Finally, health care profes-sionals will need to transform their own roles in order to share the demands imposed by chronically ill patients: old models in which doctors take responsi-bility for everything from patient education to diagnosis must give way to newer, shared ways of working together (Crabtree et al. 2010). During my obser-vations it became clear that doctors could not hope to give the same detailed, personalized care to everyone waiting to see them. The sheer number of people requiring their attention, combined with the challenge of following multiple best-practice guidelines, made this impossible. In order to survive the crush, they had to pick and choose how and where to spend their energy. When doctors are responsible for everything, some people will get almost nothing.

The women in my study wanted what we all want: good relationships with health care professionals who know us and understand us. They wanted an old-fashioned family doctor with a competent, capable staff who put them at ease. Women with broad capital were more successful at getting this need met: they accomplished it by pushing their ID clinic specialists into the role of "primary care look-alike" and co-creating healing relationships with them. But women with average capital had to make due with a rotating menu of specialists and nurses, none of whom really knew or understood them. As a result, their care—and their health—suffered.

This brings up the question of what defines a good health care professional. From the perspective of this study, it is critically important for doctors, health care professionals, and support staff to cultivate the ability to form cross-*habitus* relationships. Cultural competency training can help, but simply sharing or understanding some aspects of a culture is insufficient. Remember the story of Nini and Nadia at the clinic in chapter 6? Both shared a language and some cultural background with Dr. Sergio. But despite their overlap in background, he was unable to provide the same quality of care to Nadia as he did to Nini because he couldn't cross out of his *habitus*—he couldn't sidestep his attachment to the stigma of her substance abuse history.

There were insurmountable differences, probably class-based, between Nadia and Dr. Sergio. In cases like this, a shared language and overlapping culture alone can't bridge the gap. Good cultural competency trainers know this and urge their students not to obsess about the details of any one culture or worldview. Instead, they urge their students to cultivate the ability to bridge cultural boundaries with respect. In the long run, establishing "boundary-spanning flexibility" will result in greater success. We know this by watching Newark's resourceful women.

At the same time, clinicians and their staff are also exposed to structural violence. They, too, suffer from the effects of an impoverished urban landscape. They must identify their own coping strategies. Building a collaborative health care team that draws in local community members can help. Because local clinic and practice staff are more likely to share the problems (and *habitus*) of their patients, they may be able to respond productively under challenging but familiar circumstances. But in order for this strategy to succeed, clinic and practice staff must also receive the support and respect they need.

Finally, it is clear that average-capital women (and men) will not respond to the same kinds of initiatives that work well for broad-capital women. Health care professionals and social service agencies must work with these groups differently, reaching out with more patience and persistence to those weary of the struggle inherent in crossing boundaries. Patient navigators who specialize in helping people maneuver through the health care system may be especially invaluable for women with less exposure to middle-class institutional settings (Ferrante, Chen, and Kim 2008). Ongoing support is particularly important, since the cultural capital that can help people survive and thrive can't be absorbed in a few days or weeks. Mentorship programs that persist over time will have the greatest success.

Women with broad capital will seek out physician-partners and nurse allies to help them manage their care. They will demand information about all available treatments and value initiatives that give them access to information. They can also serve as advocates and educators who can teach others—both inexperienced, average-capital patients and their health care professionals—to cross boundaries with greater ease. Broad-capital women often thrive on the opportunity to mentor others. They may excel at training them to identify and manage the same conditions they face. They could also help clinicians learn to give better, more culturally appropriate care to their less flexible peers. If given the opportunity and ongoing structural/economic support, they could help make the health care system stronger.

Any insights I have gained spring directly from Newark's resourceful women, who managed HIV while raising families in an unforgiving and hostile environment. The deeply entrenched poverty that characterized Newark and its surrounding area is echoed in other U.S. cities like it. Under these conditions, only the most resourceful women, drawing on the greatest reserves of cultural and social capital, have any chance to thrive. The women who worked with me faced these terrible odds and extracted resources from Newark's broken safety net despite the structural violence that they faced. All had courage, and all tried to apply every resource they had to the problem of staying alive and well. But in the end, only those with extraordinary reserves of flexibility, as well as cultural and social capital, could manage Newark's compromised health care system.

This remarkable group of women helped me understand the life-and-death relationship between cultural capital and health among impoverished, chronically ill people. Their stories also point to the way theoretical concepts like Bourdieu's can illuminate social injustice, promoting change. It is my hope that the lessons for which they paid so dearly may benefit others. I am grateful for what they have taught me. I am also mindful of the legacy they have left for everyone who struggles with severe chronic illness and those who want to understand the fight. It is my dearest wish that the women who guided this project will ultimately find recognition as the teachers, mentors, and leaders they are.

Epilogue

Sorrows and Joys

Ten years have passed since I left the field. My experiences with northern New Jersey's resourceful women have shaped who I am and how I see the world. I cannot imagine who I would have become without them. My relationships with some women stayed strong, while others gradually drifted away. A few women died, and their passing broke my heart. For a long time, the memory of their deaths kept me from looking for women who had wandered out of my life. I was afraid to discover who had lived and who had died. When I finally began searching for survivors, a part of me held my breath. Who would be left alive?

To my surprise, I was able to find out what happened to every woman in this study. There were happy reunions with some women. Others talked with me over the phone. A third group had distanced themselves from the communities in which we originally met, but their caseworkers, clinicians, acquaintances, and friends knew where they were and what had happened to them in the intervening years.

In all, seven women died. Three were part of the average-capital group. Two were part of the broad-capital group. Both women in the middle group died. But the differences between these groups became most striking when I discovered who was flourishing and who was struggling. All four of the average-capital survivors grappled with health problems, depression, isolation, and/or loss. Most had become disconnected from their clinicians and some had dropped out of social service case management. None appeared particularly satisfied with their lives.

In contrast, five of the six broad-capital survivors told me (or in some cases, others) that they were happy. They reported either good health or a strong recovery from prior health problems. Some had work they loved; others lived with nurturing families. Some enjoyed both. They all pursued projects they cared about. Each one had preserved long-term healing relationships with one or

173

more health care professionals. All had stories of happiness and accomplishment to share. The sixth survivor struggled with dementia, but even she asserted that there was purpose to her life. She, too, had maintained strong, long-term relationships with several health care professionals.

Average Cultural Capital

Paquita

Halfway through my fieldwork, I came home from a summer vacation to discover that Paquita had died. Nini broke the news to me when I called to tell her I was home. When Nini had first introduced us, she had warned me that Paquita was deeply unhappy—she was trapped in an unsupportive marriage and isolated from friends and family. Even then, Nini was worried about Paquita's long-term prospects, fearing that Paquita was too isolated and depressed to help.

I was sad to learn of Paquita's death, but sadder still to think of the things she missed while she was alive: a loving, supportive network of friends and allies, high quality health care, clinicians she trusted, and a happy marriage. I wished her life had been different. I believe she deserved more than she got both from the health care system and the community in which she lived.

If there was any comfort in her story, it was in the last few months of her life. When we first met, she was living in a dark, run-down basement apartment that was barely wheelchair accessible. But a little over six months later her husband found a much nicer apartment in a better part of town. During my last few visits, Paquita showed off her new place and proudly told me how much better it was. This small bit of comfort was all I could find as I searched Paquita's life for some sign of peace.

Cristina

The last time I saw Cristina, she told me that she didn't think she had too many years left to live. She was floundering, living without a local support group. She was also anguishing over what to do about her brother, who had just moved in with her after his release from prison. He had returned to drugs, and she worried about his influence on her teenage son. As the only woman in a household of four, she did all the cooking, cleaning, and work of daily life herself. When she was sick, the work went undone. Without allies to offer her support and share her burdens, she was on her own.

Recently, I visited the clinic at which Cristina and I met. I hoped I would be able to find her. I thought that perhaps one of the clinic workers would be willing to pass along my phone number. While there, I found two people who still remembered my visits to the clinic ten years before. They gently explained that Cristina had died in 2002, about two years after our last meeting. Both remembered her well. They told me she had struggled greatly to care for herself and manage her life, right up to the end. She lost her boyfriend after he was sent to prison for a serious crime. Afterward, she continued to visit the clinic, but her health was not good. Rumors surfaced that she was back on the streets, maybe even using drugs again, although no one knew for certain. Several of the clinic's health care professionals had been very worried about her during this period.

No one knew what had happened to Cristina's son, for whom she had fought so hard. They could not tell me what had become of her brother, either. What they could say was that her death had been quick and sudden, after an acute attack of some kind. I could see the sadness on both of their faces as they told me what little they knew of her story. Cristina herself believed that she didn't have long to live. I'm sorry that she was right.

Flor

When I visited Flor's case manager, she told me that Flor had passed away many years before. Flor had lost contact with her social workers well before this happened. They had learned of her death from one of Flor's daughters. No one could tell me anything about the last stages of Flor's life or what happened to her children and family.

Juana

Juana is still living in the apartment she rented when we first met. She dropped out of the AIDS community and stopped responding to her caseworker's calls some time ago. Her social workers are concerned about the way she has isolated herself. However, she has maintained a low-key relationship with her on-again, off-again partner. Her daughter is now a young woman who attends school and works at a mall outside of Newark. Juana also has an older son who lived with his father when we first met. He and his children came to the United States to live with her for a short time, but they moved on to their own apartment shortly after.

Amelia

Amelia's husband, Pedro, died in January of 2008. For some time after I last saw the couple, he was doing well. He got a job that he enjoyed, but then fell, and this initiated a series of health problems. Later, it was discovered that he also had cancer. Amelia has also had consistent health problems since we last met. When Pedro died, her grief was made worse by the dependency she had developed on Pedro's social skills. She had depended on him to mediate between her and the world outside their neighborhood.

After Pedro's death, she withdrew even more than she had previously. Her social worker finally terminated her case because Amelia never showed up for appointments. When social workers called to check on her, Amelia said she couldn't leave the house. Her old case manager has been very concerned about Amelia's struggle to move forward and take care of herself. For example, Amelia lives in a third-floor apartment and both she and Pedro had difficulty climbing the stairs. But no matter how often her caseworker urged her to begin looking for a first-floor apartment, she refused.

Still, not all the news is bad. After Pedro's death, Amelia's mother moved in. Amelia's son married and had a baby of his own, and her daughter is in high school. Her caseworkers last saw her in January of 2009, and though she had health problems, she seemed to be holding her own.

Carlotta

Carlotta lives near the apartment in which she lived ten years ago. She has struggled with her health over the last few years, moving in and out of the hospital with frequency. She has diabetes and is currently on dialysis. Carlotta has lost weight and become very thin. Her face shows the weight of the grief and pain she has suffered. Still, she is alive. And although her health has been poor, it has not been her greatest challenge. The death of her youngest son has been her greatest cross to bear. "Why did God do this? I want to understand why. . . . I thought there would be a miracle at the last minute, something. . . . I was praying that God would take me instead—I am old and I have HIV—why not take me?" (Field note excerpt 2010).

Carlotta told me the story as her sister wept silently nearby. Her son got sick three years ago. He was diagnosed with colorectal cancer, but went into remission after his initial treatment. For a short time his health was better, but then the cancer returned, spreading to his back. He died at the age of twenty-five. Carlotta described her struggle to care for him while she herself was so weak. She told of dragging him up the stairs and fainting under his weight. Because caring for him was so hard, her sister moved in to help and remains with her still.

Carlotta's older sons have tried to console her by telling her to think about all her grandchildren, but this has not helped. Her youngest son was her closest friend and companion, and she cannot imagine life without him. "It was for him that I endured everything, this disease, everything . . . and now, why?"

Carlotta's social worker says they began working with a new holistic center specifically for her, because she really wanted the opportunity to explore CAM treatments. Ironically, Carlotta was in the hospital when the therapist was brought in, and she has missed many opportunities to work with him because of successive hospitalizations. When she finally began receiving reflexology, massage, and aromatherapy treatments, her health improved. During this period she stayed out of the hospital. But when she stopped coming to her wellness appointments—probably because of her caregiving obligations—her health took a turn for the worse. She has been readmitted to the hospital several times since. I plan to visit her the next time I return to Newark.

Nilsa

Since we last met, Nilsa has grappled with depression, weight gain, and poor health. Her social workers are concerned about her struggle with low self-esteem. Nilsa finds it difficult to take care of herself and access the resources that they and other agencies have to offer. But she does work with the recently established holistic health center. Through it, she receives reflexology and aromatherapy treatments, but takes the latest daytime appointments and forces herself to come in. Nilsa finds it is very hard to get up in the morning, and those around her have wondered if this is a symptom of depression.

On a more positive note, Nilsa finally succeeded in finding another place to live. In fact, she has moved twice since I left the field. She had hoped to find an apartment well away from drug trafficking so her younger son would find it easier to stay in recovery. However, this strategy was unsuccessful. He is currently incarcerated. Her older son, however, now has a family and a daughter of his own.

In the Middle

Luchita

It was Selma who told me what happened to Luchita. She explained that Luchita had stayed cheerful and optimistic until the very end of her life, which had come almost as soon as I stopped doing fieldwork. Selma reported that Luchita's husband was devastated by the loss of his wife and never remarried. Instead, he devoted himself to raising their children, several of whom have already begun to prosper as responsible young adults.

Selma also told me that Luchita's family was still actively involved with the church that had helped sustain them during her life. At the 2009 AIDS Day memorial service in Elizabeth, Selma introduced me to a beautiful young woman with Luchita's face. I told the girl that I had once known her mother and that I had admired her. She flashed me a brilliant, half-curious smile, as if she didn't know what to think, and dashed off to a small group of teenagers waiting in the back of the church.

Alicia

Selma, who had been one of Alicia's few close friends, told me the story of Alicia's death. She explained that after I left the field, Alicia continued to stay home, avoiding hospitals and social service agencies. Selma spoke of having to drag her friend to medical appointments and social service agencies. Eventually,

Alicia stopped taking the HIV medications she hated so much. The two women continued to live near each other during this period, so Selma was able to offer Alicia day-to-day support and assist her with chores and childcare.

Things changed when Alicia met a new man. Selma suspected him of pushing her friend into smoking pot, and she said that Alicia stopped taking care of herself during this period. Selma also told me that Alicia never told her boyfriend or her children about her HIV status. Selma described the man's anger at Alicia's funeral, when he discovered what she had withheld. He raged at Selma for keeping her friend's diagnosis a secret, but Selma answered that it was not her place to insert herself between a couple. And even if she had known that Alicia kept silent on this matter, her role as a new social service worker in the community would have bound her to confidentiality. Alicia's children, now teenagers, were also shocked at the news. Selma told me that they have yet to reconcile themselves to it, and only one of them ever speaks openly about their mother.

Broad Cultural Capital

Nerina

Around the summer of 1998, Nerina's husband died. His death was not unexpected. As a hard-drinking alcoholic, he had been in poor health for years. His on-again, off-again relationship with Nerina had been going through its usual ups and downs as he tried to control her and she sought escape his abusive bullying. When he died, she mourned his passing while recognizing that she was now free to live life on her own terms.

Over the next year and a half, Nerina was in and out of the hospital a few times, but she also reacquired her driver's license and expanded her volunteer work. When I visited her, she seemed more relaxed and centered than she had ever been in the past. She taught me to make her favorite pasta dishes and we chatted without fear of her husband. She slowly weaned herself off of methadone—which she had wanted to do for years—and felt good about her health. Her two beloved dogs kept her company, and her days often revolved around her favorite things: visiting her friends, helping out at the agency, and indulging in a little thrift shopping when possible. Nerina maintained her ties with the many social workers, doctors, and friends that she made and excitedly told me about them and her latest discoveries in complementary and alternative health care whenever we talked. No matter when I saw her, she never seemed to rest. There was always a new project or possibility on her horizon.

As my fieldwork progressed, I saw her every few weeks and we talked on the phone regularly, even when I was following other study participants. As I prepared to leave for a working vacation one spring, I got a call from one of Nerina's many friends from the HIV/AIDS service community. Nerina had gone into the hospital with PCP pneumonia a few days before. It had happened several times in the last two years, but this time, Nerina didn't recover. Her funeral would be held in a few days, and help was needed to go through her things, find a home for her dogs, and locate her wedding dress—the dress in which she wanted to be buried.

Nerina and I had seen each other only a few weeks before, and it had been a good visit. I knew she had been happy. Her death had come quickly, with little drawn-out suffering. Still, I immediately went into denial. This was not possible. Nerina had not even been sick when we had last spoken. And I was scheduled to be in Maryland, teaching both the day before and the day after her funeral. What was I going to do?

My mind shut down and I could not think. I had to call another friend, Karen, to talk me through the shock and help me make a plan. First, I would help the social worker find Nerina's wedding dress and then drive to Maryland and teach my first class. Immediately afterward I would drive back home and attend Nerina's funeral the next day. The following morning I'd get up, drive to Maryland again, and teach the second class. My friend Karen would come with me.

Once the plan had been made, I was able to relax a little. The social worker who had volunteered to sift through Nerina's things directed me as we searched through her closet for the missing wedding dress. We found it, along with a few other things Nerina had wanted to give to specific friends. Together, we made piles of clothes, books, and pieces of Nerina's life to give out to her many allies, admirers, and acquaintances. It was a good day's work, and a good way to say good-bye to a friend. When I left, the social worker gave me one of Nerina's jackets, which I wear with pride. She also gave me a large poster of Nerina herself, shining with beauty and anticipation on her wedding day.

The funeral was small but heartfelt, and Nerina would have loved the soft purple color of her cloth casket. Before I left, I said good-bye with a sad but peaceful heart. My friend had deeply enriched my life, and I had been present to honor hers.

Nini

Sometime around 1999–2000, Nini became ill. She'd been seeing a gastroenterologist for painful, persistent stomach problems ("It all started with that Cuban sandwich!" she declared ominously), but this somehow seemed worse. After multiple screenings and a confusing round of tests, she discovered that she once again faced cancer. Over the next few months, Nini lost weight, becoming very thin and frailer than I had ever seen her. But her spirit remained unchanged: every visit to her house was filled with updates about our friends and stories about her recent visits to the hospital. I heard about the successes of her (very small) jewelry business ("I sold three hundred dollars worth of jewelry to the nurse in the ER!") and learned about the latest CBO scandal. But as we laughed and gossiped, I pushed her to tell me what was really happening. What did she need? What could I do for her? As usual, she had assembled a broad range of resources and a home health aid visited regularly. Still, I worried: would this be the last time I saw her? Would this be our last visit together?

As her health improved little by little, I started to relax. She regained a little weight and began visiting her mother again more frequently. When she began scolding her teenage son and pushing me to have a baby, I knew she was feeling better. This was a relief. My formal fieldwork was coming to a close. Daily trips into Newark dwindled to once a week, and then to once every two weeks.

At the same time, I started to work on understanding the city in which Nini and her peers lived. Although I had been wandering the streets of Newark for several years, I still didn't know much about its history. I didn't understand the full scope of Newark's HIV/AIDS epidemic, nor did I know much about how city and state government had met the challenge. I only knew what I had seen and that I needed to know more. One day I wandered into Newark's public library and discovered a treasure trove: for decades, the city's librarians had been patiently clipping out a small mountain of HIV/AIDS-related articles. Most had come from the local paper, the *Star-Ledger*.

This HIV/AIDS clip file documented the earliest days of the epidemic and every decade since. It chronicled the city's initial shock and denial as men, women, and children began dying. With relentless detail, these articles recounted the political, cultural, and economic upheavals that followed in the wake of the disease. As a medical anthropologist, I had rarely worked with newspaper articles, but I understood what this file represented. Over the next few months, I began piecing together the story of HIV/AIDS in Newark by slowly working my way through photocopies and supplementing them with articles from the *New York Times* and other sources. The more I read, the angrier and more obsessed I became. Suddenly, I had a context into which to put women's stories, and it was uglier and more painful than I had ever imagined.

During this time I called and occasionally visited Nini. She was still thin, but her condition had not worsened. I told her little about what I was doing and focused on listening to her tell me about her life instead. When I was almost finished with the first draft of the chapter on Newark's history, I lost my cell phone. I should have replaced it immediately, but I was too obsessed with my work. When I took a final, flying trip to the Newark Public Library before wrapping up the draft, I thought about stopping at Nini's. I didn't have my cell phone, so I couldn't call first. Still, I knew she'd be happy to see me, even unannounced. But the day got later and later, and when I finally left the library, I decided to catch the train home and make dinner. A week or so later, I finished the draft and finally replaced my phone. Shortly after, I called Nini to tell her about what I had done.

Her son answered the phone. She told me that Nini had gone into the hospital a few weeks before after a sudden recurrence of pain. She had been in for only a few days before she died. "She didn't have her address book with her," her son told me. "She was writing names and numbers on the wall for me to call before she died. . . . I tried to call your number afterward. There was no answer."

I don't remember exactly what I said or did at that moment. I know I started crying. I think I scared Nini's son with my outburst. I did manage to ask what had happened after Nini's death—was there a funeral? Would there be a burial? Her son told me that I had missed them both.

The shock was immediate, and right away I began thinking about my last trip to the city. If I had gone to Nini's apartment that day, would I have seen her? Would I have found out that she was going into the hospital? Would she still have been alive? How long had it been since I'd called her— three weeks? Four? How could I have gone so long without checking in with her? How could I have missed her death, missed the moments when she had needed me most?

Shock gave way to depression, and depression became a kind of temporary paralysis. I could not believe what had happened. I could not believe I had missed the death of one of my dearest friends. My memory from that period is vague and shaky. I finally went to my academic advisor, who kindly suggested that I visit her grave and look for other ways to find closure for myself. Around the time of our talk, I called one of the many social workers who had been Nini's friend and told her what had happened. She told me she had been to the funeral. I asked if I could come and visit, and she graciously agreed.

When I arrived, she took me upstairs and told me what she could remember about Nini's funeral. She gave me a prayer card and talked to me until I calmed down a little. When I left, I felt a bit less shattered. In the end, I asked my religious community to help me design a brief ritual in which to say good-bye. I brought the prayer card and a few of the many small items Nini had given me: a little address book covered with Disney characters, a drink-mix package, and a costume-jewelry ring. The ritual helped me cope. Now I build an altar every year for the Day of the Dead and on it I put Nini's gifts and pictures. It is a small way in which to tell her that I miss her and that I am desperately sorry to have been absent during the days in which she needed me most.

Since that time, several friends and advisors have suggested that I shorten or even remove the chapter on Newark's history. I have always refused. I refused because that chapter is important: it tells the story of a city that sank to its knees before HIV/AIDS and the human costs of that choice. It also tells of the people who dragged the city up and forced it to meet the challenge so that Nini and her peers could have a fighting chance. But most of all, for me, it is the chapter that robbed me of the opportunity to be present at her death. For this reason, if no other, I have refused to remove it. The cost of its creation was too high.

Deborah

Over the years, Deborah and I have stayed in touch, talking and occasionally visiting each other. As I write this, she is celebrating her forty-ninth birthday. She has worked full-time at the hospital for a long time now. Deborah has moved into successively nicer apartments, and in 2002 she married her long-time boyfriend. She is actively involved in the lives of her three grandchildren, whom she loves very much. Her oldest grandchild is now a young teen! The joy that she finds in her children and grandchildren have helped her cope with the loss of both her father and brother.

Of course, Deborah has pursued a wide range of projects. She recently became board-certified in CPR, and took up photography and oil painting. She dances to salsa music every day for the pure joy of it. After twenty-seven years she finally stopped smoking in October of 2009. She says that withdrawing from nicotine was difficult, but nothing like the withdrawal experiences of her youth. Recently she volunteered for part of a children's summer camp.

Deborah's health has been up and down. She was in the hospital with pneumonia for some time, and had a benign tumor removed from her neck. Through it all, she has remained strong in her Catholic faith. Most recently, she battled shingles but refused most of the morphine her doctors have offered her. As a person in recovery, she is uncomfortable taking painkillers. Despite her own challenges, Deborah continues to act as a lay counselor to friends, colleagues, and acquaintances. She is frequently sought out by those who have experienced a loss or a trauma, and she continues to support others while facing her own challenges. I hope to offer her the same support that she has given so many others as she continues to recover.

Selma

Selma has once again become a good friend and she and I have resumed our monthly lunches at a local restaurant. Over the last ten years, she became a social worker and stayed active in the HIV/AIDS community. Selma worked for two different social service agencies and drew her partner and children into additional volunteer activities. She remains with the partner she met in the middle of my fieldwork and has continued to take in children—some related, some not—in need of good homes. Her adopted son and newborn granddaughter bring her great joy and give an important direction to her life.

The manner in which Selma prepared her children for the news that she is HIV-positive is nothing short of remarkable. When I left the field, she had already become active as a volunteer in the AIDS community. As her children got older, she drew her whole family into volunteer activities as well, telling them how important it was for them to offer acceptance and love to those living with the virus. In this way, she was also able to educate them about how to protect themselves from the virus. Because of their experiences in the AIDS community, her children were able to help one of their own peers struggling with a severe chronic illness:

> I didn't want to tell my kids before giving them the education, the 101 training. . . . It came to a point where we was doing a lot of things with the kids. We was doing a lot of things with the kids at the [AIDS Fellowship group] and they were involved in a lot of stuff. My oldest son started working for "Q" University [a pseudonym]. At sixteen he was working for them, giving speaking engagements and teaching about HIV. He was just doing it on his own, and then he found out that [I had the virus]. But it was an open door to help them understand and also it was an open door for me to tell them, in 2004, that I was HIV-positive. . . . I wanted them to know what other people was feeling . . . that it's OK to be around [people living with the virus]. That it was OK if somebody at school came to them and said, "Look, I've got a problem." As a matter of fact, one of their friends was diabetic and it was cool because even though it wasn't the virus, it was a disease that my children was helping him cope with. It was wonderful.

Recently, Selma was diagnosed with cervical cancer. She went into the hospital for a partial hysterectomy, and has healed well from this experience. She is once again going strong, and I expect to be eating many lunches with her in the future.

Celestina

While I was still in the field, Celestina and Roberto went back to Puerto Rico with her children. They moved into a small rental house near Celestina's family. She and I kept in touch over the years by mail and occasionally by phone, and I was able to visit her in 2008. As we walked around the village, she told me that shortly after she arrived, she found good health care at a local clinic and even developed a close relationship with the doctor that she and Roberto still see. She is very open about her HIV status, and all of her neighbors know about it. She is active in her community and has a broad circle of friends.

Celestina also told me a little about her work history. She always enjoyed working and was eager to look for a part-time job. After settling in, she began working part-time for a friend of a friend, a family physician who needed help organizing and managing his office. Roberto also took a job as a security guard and the two of them settled into a life that revolved around family time and part-time work. Eventually, Celestina took a short course in medical billing to learn more about office management, and eventually she became a kind of part-time office manager. This was a role that she very much enjoyed. She looks forward to taking more classes at the local community college when time and money allow.

I asked if she had ever decided to take HIV medications. She told me that she had just begun a new regimen a few months earlier. She also explained that her virus remained under control, as did Roberto's. More recently, she went into the hospital for pneumonia but recovered beautifully.

Both of her sons have grown up and each has returned to the United States to work and study. One is separated from his partner, but continues to have good relations with her. He has a son, who is the apple of Celestina's eye. He and his mother live next door to Celestina and Roberto and both of them spend a great deal of time with their first grandson. Celestina's second son is engaged to be married, and she looks forward to his wedding.

I am hopeful that Celestina and Roberto will be able to visit me this year. If not, I plan to bring my family to meet them. Thinking of their good health and flourishing family life never fails to bring joy to my heart.

Caridad

As I write, Caridad is enrolled in college and is doing very well! She is interested in pursuing a criminal justice degree. Caridad still lives in Newark. Her husband died a few years after we last spoke when a vessel burst in his brain. Because of this tragedy, Caridad and Eduardo had only a few years in which to enjoy their marriage. Eduardo's death was a shock for Caridad, as he was HIV-negative. They have one child—a little girl who is also HIV-negative. She was only two when her father died. Upon his death, Caridad was faced with the challenge of raising two young children alone as a single mother. I asked her how she did it and she said—"I don't know. I really don't know—I just did what I had to do." Her husband's family provided no support and she had to raise them all by herself.

This was very hard, but she depended on the assistance of agencies like CURA that helped her get access to both health and mental health care services. Caridad entered a long and supportive relationship with a therapist who helped her face her challenges and succeed. To this day she prizes his support and describes how he was even willing to overcome the language barrier between them in order to help her. Though she now sees another therapist, she counts him as an ally and friend. Caridad has also established a trusting relationship with a doctor, an HIV specialist whom she respects. Her T-cells are at 798, even after twenty-one years of living with the virus. For many years she was on the same drug regimen, but recently contracted diabetes, partly because of the HIV drugs. Two months ago, her physician put her on a new drug, a single pill that she takes twice a day.

Caridad's son and daughter are both flourishing. Her son is a junior attending high school. He wants to become either an FBI agent or a doctor. Caridad's daughter is in the fourth grade and is also doing well. Caridad has been seeing a new man for some time now, but has continued to stay focused on moving forward with her own goals.

In addition to attending college, Caridad was able to stop smoking and has continued to be a regular exerciser. She maintains a membership at a gym and works out at the college as well. She is fanatical about staying healthy and taking good care of herself. When I asked if she had anything else to say, she smiled and said, "For me, the sun shines every day." Then she showed me a tattoo of the sun on her ankle. Caridad's happiness exudes from her whole being, and this fills me with joy. I plan to attend her graduation ceremony, celebrating alongside her.

Gabrielle

Before I left the field, Gabrielle began struggling with HIV/AIDS-related dementia. She told me that she sometimes left her front door wide open when she left for the day, and she worried that someday she might leave the stove on. Even then, she thought it would be better if she lived with a roommate who could watch over her. As I began searching for Gabrielle, I wondered if I would find her alive. Would she even know who I was?

Last week I found several members of the HIV/AIDS service community who knew Gabrielle and remembered our work together on the Help-Seeking Pathways project. They told me that Gabrielle is indeed still alive. Her health is stable, but her dementia has worsened considerably. I asked if she had found someone to live with her and watch over her and was told that she was living near her sister, who keeps an eye on her and makes sure she is OK.

I asked one of the ladies who spoke with me to tell Gabrielle that I hope to see her again. She suggested that I write a note to Gabrielle's primary physician, asking her to pass along my request, with my phone number. I did so, and I am hoping to see my friend again soon. One of the ladies who spoke with me said that Gabrielle herself sometimes wonders aloud about her long survival. "'God must have some purpose for me,' she says." Gabrielle and I were close, and I have often wondered where she was and what happened to her. Now, I have the chance to see her again.

Julia

Julia is now living in the southern part of the state. She had a joint replacement during the ten years in which I was out of the field, but recovered afterward. An old friend says that Julia is enjoying life with her family. She described a visit she made to Julia's new home two years ago. She saw Julia again last year when Julia returned to Newark for a visit. One of Julia's prior social workers says that she hears from Julia's family every now and then, and Julia is happy.

Watching Newark Change

In 2006, Cory Booker replaced Sharpe James as mayor. His inauguration was greeted with a mix of hope and skepticism. Could he really change the tremendous economic and health disparities facing Newark's residents? In 2010, the jury is still out, but change seems to be coming. Dr. Sandra Echeverría, a social epidemiologist who has lived in Newark and conducted several studies there, sees both great challenges and cause for hope. Her analysis of Newark's mortality trends from 1960 to 2004 shows that the city still has a long way to go.

In 2004, AIDS was still the third leading cause of death for Newark's residents, despite the fact that it didn't even appear on a list of the top seven causes of death in either New Jersey or the United States. Dr Echeverría's analysis also showed that while educational achievement among residents had improved slightly, it still fell short of national levels. She also found that unemployment had doubled over the last forty years. Finally, Newark's death rates were consistently higher than those of either New Jersey or the nation. In this analysis, AIDS, diabetes, and homicide-related deaths were all shown to have a disproportionate impact on city residents (Echeverría 2007).

Still, Dr. Echeverría sees cause for hope. She points out that the mayor has partnered with celebrities like Jon Bon Jovi to call attention to Newark's problems and establish institutions that can help. At the close of 2009, Bon Jovi's Soul Foundation opened a fifty-one-unit apartment building for low-income families with special needs and those living with HIV/AIDS. HELP Genesis JBJ Soul Homes will offer North Ward residents access to community computer labs, an art gallery, and other resources. It will even have an environmentally friendly "green" roof (Simon 2009). The mayor has also created a public-private partnership to transform thirteen of Newark's parks into welcoming green spaces for sports, exercise, and leisure activities (DiIonno 2008). Changes like these give Dr. Echeverría, who conducts a local parks project of her own, hope that positive change is unfolding in Newark (S. Echeverría, pers. comm.).

Community-Based Organizations

CURA's small HIV/AIDS department is still going strong. The dedicated case managers who work there struggle for every dollar, but they continue to provide services to HIV-positive individuals who need their help. Two other Latino agencies have also consolidated their efforts and a new holistic health center has been established. The Northeast Holistic Center is funded by Ryan White grant money to offer reflexology, aromatherapy, and upper-body massage to HIV-positive individuals in the greater Newark area. A long-time local case manager described the effects of the center's treatments on her clients:

> We are seeing really positive things from this . . . but it ALL depends on what the client wants to do. Sometimes [the therapist] advises them to clean up their diet and they do. He will create immune-enhancing oils and prepare oils and lotions especially for them. It's unbelievable [how much this helps] . . . some clients can't wait five weeks for their appointments. Appointments are given every five weeks, and [he] comes to [local] agencies to meet with people. (Field note excerpt 2000)

New HIV Medications

Almost all of the women in my study wanted a simple, once-a-day HIV medication. In 2006 the FDA approved Atripla, the first of this kind. It combines three of the drugs most frequently prescribed together (Sustiva, Viread, and Emtriva) in a single, once-a-day dose. When I spoke to one of the clinic nurses who had been part of my study, she marveled at the difference Atripla made to her HIV-positive patients. "Now, it's so much easier than it used to be. . . . Do you remember how hard it was?" When I asked how she had managed to stay in such a stressful job for so many years, she laughed. "I love this job. I was here when all we had was AZT. I saw so many people die. Why wouldn't I stay, now that we have something like this to offer?"

Needle Exchange

On December 19, 2006, New Jersey became the last state in the country to legalize needle-exchange programs for IV drug users. On that day, Governor Jon Corzine signed legislation authorizing the creation of a needle-exchange pilot program. In some ways, this was the end of a bitter, decades-long battle between HIV/AIDS advocates and conservative government officials. In others, it was just another moment in the uphill battle to establish needle-exchange in Newark. When the pilot program launched in four New Jersey cities, it faced a long list of challenges, including a very tight budget and the requirement that participants carry ID cards.

From the beginning, the Newark pilot lagged behind its three sister projects in Atlantic City, Camden, and Paterson. It did not open until 2008, and when it did, it faced local opposition from those who believed that it was "enabling and increasing the use of drugs," (Kaiser 2009). As of this writing, the future of the needle-exchange program in Newark is still unclear. It has been operating on a shoestring budget since its inception (Kaiser 2008) and as the pilot drawns to a close, future funding is uncertain. How will Newark move forward on this issue? Will it break with its history and follow the lead of cities like New York and San Francisco, funding programs that keep HIV/AIDS in check? Or will it sink back into old patterns of fear, shame, and blame, allowing the disease to spread along its favorite channels once more?

February 2, 2010

REFERENCE LIST

Abraham, L. K. 1993. *Mama might be better off dead: The failure of health care in urban America.* Chicago: University of Chicago Press.

Acosta-Belén, E., and C. E. Santiago. 2006. *Puerto Ricans in the United States: A contemporary portrait.* Boulder, CO: Lynne Rienner.

Agins, B. D., K. W. Heiner, A. Bagley, I. S. Feldman, W. Ferguson, G. Camino, P. G. Weinberg, and G. S. Birkhead. 2004. Access to antiretroviral therapy during scale-up of HAART from 1996–2002: Lessons from New York state. Paper presented at the 15th International Conference on AIDS, Bangkok, Thailand.

Agnoletto, V., F. Chiaffarino, P. Nasta, R. Rossi, and F. Parazzini. 2003. Reasons for complementary therapies and characteristics of use among HIV-infected people. *International Journal of STD and AIDS* 14 (7): 482–486.

AIDS Education Global Information System. So little time . . . : An AIDS history. http://www.aegis.com/topics/timeline (accessed July 28, 2007).

AIDS Info Glossary. United States Department of Health and Human Services, http://www.aidsinfo.nih.gov/Glossary/GlossaryDefaultCenterPage.aspx (accessed April 12, 2010).

Alonso, M. A., and M. T. Koreck. 1993. Silences: "Hispanics," AIDS and sexual practices. In *The lesbian and gay studies reader,* ed. M. A. Barale, H. Abelove, and D. M. Halperin, 110–126. New York: Routledge.

Altman, L. K. 1981. Rare cancer seen in 41 homosexuals. *New York Times,* July 3.

Amaro, H. 1988. Considerations for prevention of HIV among Hispanic women. *Psychology of Women Quarterly* 12:429–443.

Anderson, W., B. O'Connor, R. R. MacGregor, and J. S. Sanford Schwartz. 1993. Patient use and assessment of conventional and alternative therapies for HIV infection and AIDS. *AIDS* 7 (4): 561–565.

Arici, C., D. Ripamonti, V. Ravasio, F. Maggiolo, M. Rizzi, and M.G. Finazzi. 2001. Long-term clinical benefits of highly active anti-retroviral therapy in advanced HIV-1 infection, even in patients without immune reconstitution. *International Journal of STD and AIDS* 12 (9): 573–581.

Aun, F. J. 1990. 'Day of hope' sheds light on AIDS epidemic. *Star-Ledger* (Newark), December 2.

Baer, H., M. Singer, and I. Susser. 1997. *Medical anthropology and the world system: A critical perspective.* Westport, CT: Bergin & Garvey.

Baker, S. S. 2002. *Understanding mainland Puerto Rican poverty.* Philadelphia: Temple University Press.

Barkan, S. E., S. L. Melnick, S. Preston-Martin, K. Weber, L. A. Kalish, P. Miotti, M. Young, R. Greenblatt, H. Sacks, and J. Feldman. 1998. The women's interagency HIV study. *Epidemiology* 9 (2): 117–125.

Berger, M. T. 2004. *Workable sisterhood: The political journey of stigmatized women with HIV/AIDS*. Princeton: Princeton University Press.

Bergmann, L. 2008. *Getting ghost: Two young lives and the struggle for the soul of an American city*. New York: The New Press.

Bernard, H. R. 1994. *Research methods in anthropology: Qualitative and quantitative approaches*. 2nd ed. Thousand Oaks, CA: Sage Publications.

Boodman, S. G. 1989. Up against it: In Newark a public hospital fights the twin plagues of AIDS and drugs. *Washington Post*, September 5.

Boon, H., M. Verhoef, D. O'Hara, and B. Findlay. 2004. From parallel practice to integrative health care: A conceptual framework. *BMC Health Services Research* 4 (15). http://www.biomedcentral.com/1472–6963/4/15 (accessed January 31, 2010).

Bourdieu, P. 1986. The forms of capital. In *Handbook of theory and research for the sociology of education*, ed. J. G. Richardson, 241–258. New York: Greenwood Press.

Bourgois, P. 2003. *In search of respect: Selling crack in El Barrio*. Cambridge: Cambridge University Press.

Bowser, B. P., E. Quimby, and M. Singer, eds. 2007. *When communities assess their AIDS epidemics: Results of rapid assessment of HIV/AIDS in eleven U.S. cities*. New York: Lexington Books.

Bury, J., V. Morrison, and S. McLachlan, eds. 1992. *Working with women and AIDS: Medical, social, and counseling issues*. London: Tavistock/Routledge.

Byrd, F. W. 1983. 'Invisibility' casts pall on Puerto Rican population: Report claims business, government ignore Newark's Hispanic residents. *Star-Ledger* (Newark), June 27.

Byrd, F. W. 1988a. AIDS test controversy won't halt Newark prostitution crackdown. *Star-Ledger* (Newark), January 24.

Byrd, F. W. 1988b. Newark hospitals hope to open AIDS care facility by year's end. *Star-Ledger* (Newark), April 8.

Byrd, F. W. 1988c. Long-time Newarkers make up most cases. *Star-Ledger* (Newark), January 28.

Byrd, F. W. 1988d. James pushes 'long-term care' facility in Newark for AIDS sufferers: Mayor sees state funds needed after meeting with hospital execs. *Star-Ledger* (Newark), February 2.

Byrd, F. W. 1988e. Newark's grim reaper: AIDS the fifth-leading cause of death as the toll doubles. *Star-Ledger* (Newark), March 8.

Byrd, F. W. 1988f. Forum mobilizes Newark group against AIDS: Mayor outlines steps being taken to combat disease, rumors, fears. *Star-Ledger* (Newark), March 13.

Calabrese, C., C. A. Wenner, C. Reeves, P. Turet, and L. J. Standish. 1998. Treatment of human immunodeficiency virus-positive patients with complementary and alternative medicine: A survey of practitioners. *Journal of Alternative and Complementary Medicine* 4 (3): 281–287.

Campbell, C. A. 2006. The youngest patients keep a pioneering doctor busy. *AIDS at 25*, pt.3. *Star-Ledger* (Newark), July 18.

CDC. *See* Centers for Disease Control and Prevention.

Centers for Disease Control and Prevention. 2009. HIV statistics and surveillance: Basic statistics. http://www.cdc.gov/hiv/topics/surveillance/basic.htm (current as of February 26, 2009; accessed July 3, 2009).

Chambré, S. M. 2006. *Fighting for our lives: New York's AIDS community and the politics of disease*. New Brunswick, NJ: Rutgers University Press.

CHASS. *See* Community Health and Social Services Center.

Chu, S. Y., J. W. Buehler, and R. L. Berkelman. 1990. Impact of the human immunodeficiency virus epidemic on mortality in women of reproductive age, United States. *Journal of the American Medical Association* 264 (2): 225–229.

Clatts, M. 1994. Poverty, drug use and AIDS: Converging issues in the life stories of women in Harlem. In *Wings of gauze: Women of color and the experience of health and illness*, ed. B. Bair and S. Cayliff, 328–339. Detroit: Wayne State University Press.

Community Health and Social Services Center. http://www.chasscenter.org/present.htm (accessed August 15, 2009).

Connecticut Department of Public Health. 2002. *Epidemiologic profile of HIV and AIDS*. Hartford: Connecticut Department of Public Health.

Connors, M. 1996. Sex, drugs, and structural violence. In *Women, poverty, and AIDS: Sex, drugs, and structural violence*, eds. P. Farmer, M. Connors, and J. Simmons, 91–123. Monroe, ME: Common Courage Press.

Corea, G. 1992. *The invisible epidemic: The story of women and AIDS*. New York: HarperCollins.

Correll, P. K., M. G. Law, A. M. McDonald, D. A. Cooper, and J. M. Kaldor. 1998. HIV disease progression in Australia in the time of combination antiretroviral therapies. *Medical Journal of Australia* 169 (9): 469–472.

Crabtree, B. F., P. A. Nutting, W. L. Miller, K. C. Stange, E. E. Stewart, and C. R. Jaén. 2010. Summary of the national demonstration project and recommendations for the patient-controlled medical home. *Annals of Family Medicine* 8 (Suppl. no. 1): 580–590.

Cruz, J. E. 2003. Unfulfilled promise: Puerto Rican politics and poverty. *Centro Journal* 15 (1): 153–175.

CURA. Background: CURA's history. http://www.curainc.org/history.htm (accessed July 28, 2007).

Curtis, R., A. Conde, M. Irizarry, and C. Wolf. 2007. Responding to the AIDS crisis in Newark, New Jersey. In *When communities assess their AIDS epidemics: Results of rapid assessment of HIV/AIDS in eleven U.S. cities*, ed. B. P. Bower, E. Quimby, and M. Singer, 29–45. Lanham, MD: Lexington Books.

de la Torre, A., R. Friis, H. Hunter, and L. Garcia. 1996. The health insurance status of U.S. Latino women: A profile from the 1982–1984 HHANES [Hispanic Health and Nutrition Examination Survey]. *American Journal of Public Health* 86 (4): 533–537.

de Zalduando, B., and J. M. Bernard. 1995. Meanings and consequences of sexual-economic exchange: Gender, poverty, and sexual risk behavior in urban Haiti. In *Conceiving sexuality: Approaches to research in a postmodern world*, ed. R. Parker and J. Gagnon, 157–180. New York: Routledge.

DiIonno, M. 2008. Big dreams for Newark's broken parks. *NJ Voices: Opinions from New Jersey*. http://blog.nj.com/njv_mark_diionno/2008/03/big_dreams_for_newarks_broken.html (accessed January 31, 2010).

Dorn, N., S. Henderson, and N. South, eds. 1992. *AIDS: Women, drugs and social care*. London: Falmer Press.

Douard, J., and J. D. Durham. 1993. HIV-infected women and children: Social and ethical perspectives. In *Women, children and HIV/AIDS*, ed. F. L. Cohen and J. Durham, 228–240. New York: Springer.

Duggan, J., W. S. Peterson, M. Schultz, S. Khuder, and J. Chakravarty. 2001. Use of complementary and alternative therapies in HIV-infected patients. *AIDS Patient Care Studies* 15 (3): 159–167.

Echeverría, S. 2007. Mortality trends for Newark, N.J.: 1960–2004. Monograph, UMDNJ School of Public Health, Institute for the Elimination of Health Disparities.

Elisabeth (no surname given). 1987. Being positive is positive. In *AIDS: The women*, ed. I. Reider and P. Ruppert, 81–87. San Francisco: Cleis Press.

Elmelech, Y., and H. H. Lu. 2004. Race, ethnicity, and the gender poverty gap. *Social Science Research* 33:158–182.

Fadiman, A. 1997. *The spirit catches you and you fall down: A Hmong child, her American doctors, and the collision of two cultures.* New York: Noonday Press.

Fairfield, K. M., D. M. Eisenberg, R. B. Davis, H. Libman, and R. S. Phillips. 1998. Patterns of use, expenditures, and perceived efficacy of complementary and alternative therapies in HIV-infected patients. *Archives of Internal Medicine* 158:2257–2264.

Farmer, P., M. J. D. Good, and S. Lindenbaum. 1993. Women, poverty, and AIDS: An introduction. *Culture, Medicine, and Psychiatry* 17 (4): 387–397.

Farmer, P., J. Simmons, and M. Connors, eds. 1996. *Women, poverty, and AIDS: Sex, drugs, and structural violence.* Monroe, ME: Common Courage Press.

Ferrante, J., P. Chen, and S. Kim. 2008. The effect of patient navigation on time to diagnosis, anxiety, and satisfaction in urban minority women with abnormal mammograms: A randomized controlled trial. *Journal of Urban Health* 85 (1): 114–124.

Fiscella, K., P. Franks, M. R. Gold, and C. M. Clancy. 2000. Inequality in quality: Addressing socioeconomic, racial, and ethnic disparities in health care. *Journal of the American Medical Association* 283 (19): 2579–2584.

Frye, V., M. H. Latka, Y. F. Wu, E. E. Valverde, A. R. Knowlton, K. R. Knight, J. H. Arnstein, and A. O'Leary. 2007. Intimate partner violence perpetration against main female partners among HIV-positive male injection drug users. *Journal of Acquired Immune Deficiency Syndromes* 46 (Suppl. no. 2): S101–S109.

Furin, J. 1995. Becoming my own doctor: Gay men, AIDS, and alternative therapy use in West Hollywood, California. PhD diss., University of California, Los Angeles.

Glanz, K., R. T. Croyle, V. Chollette, and V. Pinn. 2003. Cancer-related health disparities in women. *American Journal of Public Health* 93 (2): 292–298.

Gluck, G. H. 1987. Total community effort needed to combat AIDS. *Star-Ledger* (Newark), July 27.

Goosby, E. 2007. Preface to *When communities assess their AIDS epidemics: Results of rapid assessment of HIV/AIDS in eleven U.S. cities*, ed. B. P. Bowser, E. Quimby, and M. Singer, vii–ix. Lanham, MD: Lexington Books.

Gore-Felton, C., M. Vosvick, R. Power, C. Koopman, E. Ashton, M. Bachman, D. Israelson, and D. Spiegel. 2003. Alternative therapies: A common practice among men and women living with HIV. *Journal of the Association of Nurses in AIDS Care* 14 (3): 17–27.

Greenblatt, R., P. Bacchetti, S. Barkan, M. Augenbraun, S. Silver, R. Delapenha, P. Garcia, U. Mathur, P. Miotti, and D. Burns. 1999. Lower genital tract infections among HIV-infected and high-risk uninfected women: Findings of the women's interagency HIV study (WIHS). *Sexually Transmitted Diseases* 26 (3): 143–151.

Greene, K. B., J. Berger, C. Reeves, A. Moffatt, L. J. Standish, and C. Calabrese. 1999. Most frequently used alternative and complementary therapies and activities by participants in the AMCOA study. *Journal of the Association of Nurses in AIDS Care* 10 (3): 60–73.

Groves, B. 1994. Whitman urges HIV test for all pregnant women. *Hackensack (NJ) Record*, April 6.

Hajet, A., J. Lucas, and R. Kingston. 2000. Health outcomes among Hispanic subgroups: Data from the national health interview survey, 1992–1995. *Advance Data*, no.310:1–14.

Hammonds, E. 1992. Missing persons: African American women, AIDS and the history of disease. *Radical America* 24 (2).

Hancock, E. L. 2002. AIDS is just a four letter word: An ethnographic study of theodicy and the social construction of HIV/AIDS in Newark, New Jersey. PhD diss., Drew University.

Hayden, T. 1967. *Rebellion in Newark; official violence and ghetto response*. New York: Vintage Books.

Health Resources and Services Administration. The Ryan White HIV/AIDS program. http://hab.hrsa.gov/about/ (accessed January 22, 2008).

Health Resources and Services Administration. 2006. Ryan White Care Act fact sheet, July 2006.

Heimer, R., S. Clair, L. Grau, R. Bluthenal, P. Marshall, and M. Singer. 2002. Hepatitis-associated knowledge is low and risks are high among HIV-aware injection drug users in three U.S. cities. *Addiction* 97:1277–1282.

Heimer, R., L. Grau, E. Curtin, K. Khoshnood, and M. Singer. 2007. Assessment of HIV testing of urban injection drug users: Implications for expansion of HIV testing and prevention efforts. *American Journal of Public Health* 97 (1): 110–116.

Henderson, S. 1992. Living with the virus: Perspectives from HIV-positive women in London. In *AIDS: Women, drugs and social care*, ed. N. Dorn, S. Henderson, and N. South, 7–24. London: Falmer Press.

Henry J. Kaiser Family Foundation. The global HIV/AIDS timeline. http://www.kff.org/hivaids/timeline/hivtimeline.cfm (accessed August 18, 2009).

Henry J. Kaiser Family Foundation. 2007. HIV/AIDS epidemic in the United States. HIV/AIDS Policy Fact Sheet, no. 3029–07. http://www.kff.org.

Henry J. Kaiser Family Foundation. 2008. Kaiser Health News' daily report, February 26. http://www.kaiserhealthnews.org/daily-reports/2008/february/26/dr00050598.aspx?referrer=search (accessed February 2, 2010).

Henry J. Kaiser Family Foundation. 2009. Kaiser Health News' daily report, April 15. http://www.kaiserhealthnews.org/daily-reports/2009/april/15/dr00058011.aspx?referrer=search (accessed February 2, 2010).

Herman, M. 2005. *Fighting in the streets: Ethnic succession in 20th century America*. New York: Peter Lang.

Herman, M. 2007. Riots–1967. http://www.67riots.rutgers.edu/n_index.htm (accessed July 25, 2007).

Herron, J. 1993. *Afterculture: Detroit and the humiliation of history*. Detroit: Wayne State University Press.

HHS. *See* U.S. Department of Health and Human Services.

Holmes, W. C., and J. L. Pace. 2002. HIV-seropositive individuals' optimistic beliefs about prognosis and relation to medication and safe sex adherence. *Journal of General Internal Medicine* 17: 677–683.

HRSA. *See* Health Resources and Services Administration.

HUD. *See* U.S. Department of Housing and Urban Development.

Ives, N. J., B. G. Gazzard, and P. J. Eastbrook. 2001. The changing pattern of AIDS-defining illnesses with the introduction of highly active anti-retroviral therapy (HAART) in a London clinic. *Journal of Infection* 42 (2): 134–139.

John, G., and J. Kreiss. 1996. Mother-to-child transmission of human immunodeficiency virus type I. *Epidemiologic Reviews* 18 (2): 149–157.

Johnson, D., and S. Ross. Timeline: AIDS epidemic: Key events, important people, activism and breakthroughs. http://www.infoplease.com/spot/aidstimeline1.html (accessed July 28, 2007).

Jones, J. H. 1981. *Bad blood: The Tuskegee syphilis experiment: A tragedy of race and medicine*. New York: Free Press.

Kaiser. *See* Henry J. Kaiser Family Foundation.

Kim, Y. J., N. Peragallo, and B. DeForge. 2006. Predictors of participation in an HIV risk reduction intervention for socially deprived Latino women: A cross sectional cohort study. *International Journal of Nursing Studies* 43:527–534.

King, S., director. 1987. Newark: The slow road back. NJCore: New Jersey Digital Repository. http://fdr.njedge.net/njvid/showvideo.php?pid=njcore:16599 (accessed April 12, 2010).

King, S., director. 2007. Due Process special: Newark rebellion 40th anniversary. New Jersey Network Public Television and Radio documentary. Description at http://www.njn.net/television/njnseries/dueprocess/2007season/newarkrebellion.html (accessed April 12, 2010).

Kleinman, A. 1980. *Patients and healers in the context of culture: An exploration of the borderland between anthropology, medicine, and psychiatry.* Berkeley: University of California Press.

Kleinman, A. 1988. *The illness narratives: Suffering, healing and the human condition.* New York: Basic Books.

Kneisl, C. R. 1993. Psychosocial and economic concerns of women affected by HIV infection. In *Women, children, and HIV/AIDS*, ed. F. L. Cohen and J. Durham, 241–250. New York: Springer.

Knippels, H. M., and J. J. Weiss. 2001. Use of alternative medicine in a sample of HIV-positive gay men: An exploratory study of prevalence and user characteristics. *AIDS Care* 12:435–446.

Kukla, B. 1993. Zoning board votes for AIDS care facility at nursing home. *Star-Ledger* (Newark), February 15.

Kukla, B. 1995. Battling a viral enemy: Residents on the front lines in struggle against AIDS. *Star Ledger* (Newark), March 20.

Kurth, A. 1993. An overview of women and HIV disease. In *Until the cure: Caring for women with HIV*, ed. A. Kurth, 1–18. New Haven, CT: Yale University Press.

LaGuardia, K. D. 1991. AIDS and reproductive health: Women's perspectives. In *AIDS and women's reproductive health*, ed. L. C. Chen, J. S. Amor and S. J. Segal, 17–25. New York: Plenum Press.

LaKosky, P., E. Ward, and L. Ouellet. 2007. AIDS health emergency in Chicago. In *When communities assess their AIDS epidemics: Results of rapid assessment of HIV/AIDS in eleven US cities*, ed. B. P. Bowser, E. Quimby, and M. Singer, 47–63. Lanham, MD: Lexington Books.

Larson, P. D. 2009. Illness behavior. In *Chronic illness: Impact and intervention*, ed. P. D. Larson and I. Lubkin, 25–41. Sudbury, MA: Jones and Bartlett Publishers.

Latino Family Services. Mission statement. http://latinofamilyservices.org/Welcome.aspx (accessed August 15, 2009).

Leusner, D. 1990a. Health officials warn against narrow AIDS focus. *Star-Ledger* (Newark), July 15.

Leusner, D. 1990b. Jersey AIDS rate rises among heterosexuals. *Star-Ledger* (Newark), September 21.

Lewis, D. K. 1993. Living with the threat of AIDS: Perceptions of health and risk among African American iv drug users. In *Wings of gauze: Women of color and the experience of health and illness*, ed. B. Bair and S. Cayliff, 312–327. Detroit: Wayne State University Press.

Lewis, D. K., and J. K. Waters. 1988. Human immunodeficiency virus seroprevalence in female intravenous drug users: The puzzle of black women's risk. *Social Science and Medicine* 29 (9): 1071–1076.

López, M. E. 2007. Investigating the investigators: An analysis of the Puerto Rican study. *Centro Journal* 19 (2): 61–85.

Lorig, K. 2002. Partnerships between expert patients and physicians. *The Lancet* 359:814–815.

LSU Law Center.1993. The History of AIDS and ARC (by E. P. Richards). http://biotech .law.lsu.edu/Books/lbb/x590.htm#fnB132 (accessed November 28, 2007).

Loue, S., and M. Sajatovic. 2006. Spirituality, coping, and HIV risk and prevention in a sample of severely mentally ill Puerto Rican women. *Journal of Urban Health* 83 (6): 1168–1182.

MacLeod, J. 1995. *Ain't no makin' it: Aspirations and attainment in a low-income neighborhood.* Boulder, CO: Westview Press.

Maisels, L., J. Steinberg, and C. Tobias. 2001. An investigation of why eligible patients do not receive HAART. *AIDS Patient Care and STDs* 15 (4): 185–191.

Massara, E. B. 1989. *Que gordita: A study of weight among women in a Puerto Rican community.* New York: AMS Press.

Mays, V., and S. Cochran. 1988. Issues in the perception of AIDS risk and risk reduction activities by black and Hispanic/Latina women. *American Psychologist* 4:949–957.

McLaughlin, J. 1992a. Women with AIDS finding help at a clinic founded just for them. *Star-Ledger* (Newark), March 2.

McLaughlin, J. 1992b. The AIDS trenches: Educators brave violence to help addicts. *Star-Ledger* (Newark), March 4.

Mikhail, I. S., R. Diclemente, S. Person, S. Davies, E. Elliot, G. Wingood, and P. Jolly. 2004. Association of complementary and alternative medicines with HIV clinical disease among a cohort of women living with HIV/AIDS. *Journal of Acquired Immune Deficiency Syndromes* 37 (3): 1415–1422.

Miller, B., W. Downs, and M. Testa. 1993. Interrelationship between victimization experiences and women's alcohol use. *Journal of Studies on Alcohol.* Suppl. no. 11:109–117.

Miller, J. 1993. "Your life is on the line every night you're on the streets": Victimization and resistance among street prostitutes. *Humanity and Society* 17 (4): 422–446.

Moore, R. D. 1999. Anemia and human immunodeficiency virus disease in the area of highly active anti-retroviral therapy. *Seminars in Hematology* 37 (Suppl. no. 6): 18–23.

Mosack, K., M. Abbott, M. Singer, M. Meeks, and L. Rohena. 2005. "If I didn't have HIV, I'd be dead now": Illness narratives of drug users living with HIV/AIDS. *Qualitative Health Research* 15 (5): 586–605.

Mumford, K. 2007. *Newark : A history of race, rights, and riots in America.* New York: New York University Press.

Murphy, J. 1991. Substance abuse and serious child mistreatment. *Child Abuse and Neglect* 15:197–211.

Narvaez, A. A. 1987. Newark hospitals seek unit for AIDS treatment. *New York Times*, July 21.

Narvaez, A. A. 1988. Newark moves to test for AIDS virus. *New York Times*, January 7.

National Public Radio. 2007. Examining the Newark riots 40 years later. Recorded interview with Junius Williams and Max Herman. NPR News and Notes, July 12, 2007. http://www.npr.org/templates/story/story.php?storyId=11918120 (accessed April 13, 2010).

Needle, R., R. Trotter, M. Singer, C. Bates, B. Page, D. Metzger, and I. Marcelin. 2003. Rapid assessment of the HIV/AIDS crisis in racial and ethnic minority communities: An approach for timely community interviews. *American Journal of Public Health* 93 (6).

NEMA Planning Council. *See* Newark Eligible Metropolitan Area HIV Health Services Planning Council.

Newark Eligible Metropolitan Area HIV Health Services Planning Council. Newark EMA health services planning council FAQ. http://www.newarkema.org/content/FAQ.html (accessed January 22, 2008).

New Jersey Department of Health. 1994. State of New Jersey Department of Health fact sheet.

New Jersey Women and AIDS Network. What we're about. http://www.njwan.org/about.html (accessed November 12, 2007).

NJWAN. *See* New Jersey Women and AIDS Network.

NPR. *See* National Public Radio.

Oakley, A. 1989. Women's studies in British sociology: To end at our beginning? *British Journal of Sociology* 40 (3).

Osmond, M. W., K. G. Wambach, D. F. Harrison, J. Byers, P. Levine, A. Imershein, and D. M. Quadagno. 1992. The multiple jeopardy of race, class, and gender for AIDS risk among women. *Gender and Society* 7 (1): 99–120.

Parks, B. 2007a. Crossroads, pt.1: Before 1967, a gathering storm. *Star-Ledger* (Newark), July 8.

Parks, B. 2007b. Crossroads, pt. 2: 5 days that changed a city. *Star-Ledger* (Newark), July 9.

Parks, B. 2007c. Crossroads, pt. 3: After the riots, change is slow to come. *Star Ledger* (Newark), July 10.

Patrick, L. 2000. Nutrients and HIV: Part three—n-acetylcysteine, alpha-lipoic acid, 1-glutamine, and 1-carnitive. *Alternative Medicine Review* 5 (4): 290–305.

Patterson, M. J. 1993. Plainfield man's organization helps others learn to live with HIV, AIDS. *Star-Ledger* (Newark), July 18.

Patterson, M. J. 1994. Study launched in Newark finds drug limits AIDS transmission to unborn: Findings on AZT called "exciting" for HIV-positive pregnant women. *Star-Ledger* (Newark), February 22.

Patton, C. 1994. *Inventing AIDS.* New York: Routledge.

Pawluch, D., R. Cain, and J. Gillett. 2001. Lay constructions of HIV and complementary therapy use. *Social Science and Medicine* 51 (2): 251–264.

Peet, J. 1987a. Kids with AIDS: Jersey struggles with deadly legacy. *Star-Ledger* (Newark), December 20.

Peet, J. 1987b. The innocents: Seeking answers for children with AIDS. *Star-Ledger* (Newark), December 21.

Peet, J. 1987c. A dedicated few ease the pain of abandoned children with AIDS. *Star-Ledger* (Newark), December 22.

Peet, J., and J. Whitlow. 1987. AIDS toll forecast doubled. *Star-Ledger* (Newark), November 5.

Perez, S. 1994. At the margins. *Spectrum: The Journal of State Government* 67 (3): 41.

Phipps, J. 1989. Speaking out on AIDS: Residents, officials testify at congressional hearing. *Star-Ledger* (Newark), March 27.

Porambo, R., W. Sloat, and F. Bruning. 2007. *No cause for indictment: An autopsy of Newark.* New York: Melville House.

Rees, L. 2001. Integrated medicine. *British Medical Journal* 322:119–120.

Richardson, D. 1988. *Women and AIDS.* New York: Methuen.

Romero, G., L. Arguelles, and A. M. Rivero. 1993. Latinas and HIV infection/AIDS: Reflections on impacts, dilemmas and struggles. In *Wings of gauze: Women of color and the experience of health and illness,* ed. B. Bair and S. Cayliff, 340–352. Detroit: Wayne State University Press.

Romero, M. 1993. The use of women's culture in AIDS outreach. In *Wings of gauze: Women of color and the experience of health and illness,* ed. B. Bair and S. Cayliff, 353–363. Detroit: Wayne State University Press.

Romero-Daza, N., M. Weeks, and M. Singer. 2003. "Nobody gives a damn if I live or die": Violence, drugs, and street-level prostitution in inner-city Hartford, Connecticut. *Medical Anthropology* 22:233–259.

Romero-Daza, N., M. Weeks, and M. Singer. 2005. Conceptualizing the impact of indirect violence on HIV risk among women involved in street-level prostitution. *Aggression and Violent Behavior* 10:153–170.

Rosenthal, T. 2008. The medical home: Growing evidence to support a new approach to primary care. *Journal of the American Board of Family Medicine* 21 (5): 427–440.

Rudolph, R. 1993. Judge upholds AIDS panel firings but blasts both James and foes. *Star-Ledger* (Newark), June 8.

Sanabria, R. 2004. "Vida/SIDA: A grassroots response to AIDS in Chicago's Puerto Rican community." *Convergence* 37 (4): 37–42.

Schulte, L. 1985a. Jersey's prisons lead nation in the incidence of AIDS-infected inmates. *Star-Ledger* (Newark), February 17.

Schulte, L. 1985b. Newark minister plans shelter for AIDS victims. *Star-Ledger* (Newark), September 9.

Schwaneberg, R. 1989. One in 200 Jersey newborns tests positive for AIDS virus. *Star-Ledger* (Newark), February 10.

Scott, J. G., D. Cohen, B. DiCicco-Bloom, W. Miller, K. Stange, and B. Crabtree. 2008. Understanding healing relationships in primary care. *Annals of Family Medicine* 6 (4): 315–322. http://www.peh-med.com/content/4/1/11 (accessed April 13, 2010).

Scott, J. G., R. G. Scott, W. L. Miller, K. Stange, and B. F. Crabtree. 2009. Healing relationships and the existential philosophy of Martin Buber. *Philosophy, Ethics and Humanities in Medicine* 4:11.

Sharff, J. W. 1998. *King Kong on 4th street: Families and the violence of poverty on the Lower East Side.* Boulder, CO: Westview Press.

Shayne, L., and B. J. Kaplan. 1991. Double victims: Poor women and AIDS. *Women and Health* 17:21–37.

Siegel, K., E. Schrimshaw, and H. M. Lekas. 2006. Diminished sexual activity, interest, and feelings of attractiveness among HIV-infected women in two eras of the AIDS epidemic. *Archives of Sexual Behavior* 35:437–449.

Simon, S. 2009. Jon Bon Jovi helps open HELP Genesis JBJ Soul Homes in Newark. *Star-Ledger (Newark) Videos*, http://videos.nj.com/star-ledger/2009/12/jon_bon_jovi_helps_open_help_g.html (posted December 8, 2009).

Singer, M. 1994. AIDS and the health crisis of the U.S. urban poor: The perspective of critical medical anthropology. *Social Science and Medicine* 39 (7): 931–948.

Singer, M. 1996. A dose of drugs, a touch of violence, a case of AIDS: Conceptualizing the SAVA syndemic. *Free Inquiry in Creative Sociology* 24 (2): 99–110.

Singer, M., and H. Baer. 2007. *Introducing medical anthropology: A discipline in action.* Lanham, MD: AltaMira Press.

Singer, M., and J. Eiserman. 2007. Twilight's last gleaning: Rapid assessment of late night HIV risk in Hartford, CT. In *When communities assess their AIDS epidemics: Results of rapid assessment of HIV/AIDS in eleven U.S. cities*, ed. B. P. Bowser, E. Quimby, and M. Singer, 193–207. Lanham, MD: Lexington Books.

Singer, M., G. Scott, S. Wilson, D. Easton, and M. Meeks. 2001. "War stories": AIDS prevention and the street narratives of drug users. *Qualitative Health Research* 11 (5): 589–611.

Singer, M., J. Simmons, M. Duke, and L. Broomhall. 2001. The challenges of street research on drug use, violence, and AIDS risk. *Addiction Research and Theory* 9 (4): 365–402.

Singer, M., and M. Weeks. 1996. Preventing AIDS in communities of color: Anthropology and social prevention. *Human Organization* 55 (4): 488–492.

Singer, M., and M. Weeks. 2005. The Hartford model of AIDS practice/research collaboration. In *Community interventions and AIDS*, ed. E. J. Trickett and W. Pequegnat, 153–175. New York: Oxford University Press.

Smedley, B., A. Stith, and A. R. Nelson. 2003. *Unequal treatment: Confronting racial and ethnic disparities in health care.* Washington, D.C: National Academies Press.

Social Security Administration. 1995a. *Social Security Disability programs*, publication no. 05–10057. Washington, D.C.: U.S. Government Printing Office.

Social Security Administration. 1995b. *Social Security Disability programs can help*, publication no. 1995–387–00020006. Washington, D.C.: U.S. Government Printing Office.

Social Security Administration. 1997. *SSI in New Jersey*, publication no. 05–11148. Washington, D.C.: U.S. Government Printing Office.

Social Security Administration. n.d. *Disability benefits for people living with HIV infection fact sheet* (collected circa 1997).

Solomon, L., M. Stein, C. Flynn, P. Shuman, E. Schoenbaum, J. Moore, S. Holmberg, and N. M. H. Graham. 1998. Health services use by urban women with or at risk for HIV-1 infection: The HIV epidemiology research study (HERS). *Journal of Acquired Immune Deficiency Syndromes* 17 (3): 253–261.

Soto, M. 1995. Study finds "alarming" numbers of Newark-area women with AIDS. *Star-Ledger* (Newark), August 17.

South, S. J., K. Crowder, and E. Chavez. 2005. Exiting and entering high poverty neighborhoods: Latinos, black, and Anglos compared. *Social Forces* 84 (2): 873–900.

Sparber, A., J. C. Wootton, L. Bauer, G. Curt, D. Eisenberg, and T. Levin. 2000. Use of complementary medicine by adult patients participating in HIV/AIDS clinical trials. *Journal of Alternative and Complementary Medicine* 6 (5): 415–422.

SSA. *See* Social Security Administration.

Star-Ledger (Newark). 1987. Newark sites targeted as AIDS care centers. December 20.

Star-Ledger (Newark). 1990. Florio orders speeded approval process for AIDS home care facilities. December 18.

Star-Ledger (Newark). 1993. Grants are awarded for AIDS programs. July 20.

Standish, L. J., K. B. Greene, S. Bain, C. Reeves, F. Sanders, and R. C. Wines. 2001. Alternative medicine use in HIV-positive men and women: Demographics, utilization patterns and health status. *AIDS Care* 13 (2): 197–208.

Stewart, A. 1990. State pledges to continue AIDS program after foundation funds run out. *Star-Ledger* (Newark), September 6.

Thomas, J. 1993. Newark is portrait of AIDS' future. *Chicago Tribune*, December 12.

Thomas, S., and S. C. Quinn. 1991. Tuskegee syphilis study, 1932–1972: Implications for HIV education and AIDS risk education programs in the black community. *American Journal of Public Health* 8 (11): 1498–1505.

Thorne, S., B. Paterson, C. Russell, and A. Schulze. 2002. Complementary/alternative medicine in chronic illness as informed self-care decision making. *International Journal of Nursing Studies* 39:671–683.

Underdue, T. 1991. Not enough for AIDS: Advocates say little being done to educate, fund programs. *Star-Ledger* (Newark), November 8.

Union County HIV Consortium. n.d. Union County HIV Consortium Resource Center. Flyer.

U.S. Department of Health and Human Services. 2005. Side effects of anti-HIV medications: Health information for patients. AIDS Info Fact Sheet. http://aidsinfo.nih.gov/

contentfiles/SideEffectAnitHIVMeds_cbrochure_en.pdf (current as of October 2005; accessed April 13, 2010).

U.S. Department of Housing and Urban Development. Housing opportunities for persons with AIDS (HOPWA) program. http://www.hud.gov/offices/cpd/aidshousing/programs/ (current as of January 18, 2008; accessed January 22, 2008).

Walker, S. T. 1993a. Newark mayor ready to shuffle HIV council. *Star-Ledger* (Newark), April 9.

Walker, S. T. 1993b. Official acts to streamline the processing of funds used to fight AIDS. *Star-Ledger* (Newark), April 17.

Walker, S. T. 1993c. Newark improving distribution of AIDS funds. *Star-Ledger* (Newark), May 7.

Watstein, S. B., and R. Laurich. 1991. *AIDS and women: A sourcebook.* Phoenix, AZ: Oryx Press.

Weeks, M., S. Clair, M. Singer, K. Radda, J. Schensul, S. Wilson, and G. Knight. 2001. High risk drug use sites, meaning and practice: Implications for AIDS prevention. *Journal of Drug Issues* 31 (1): 781–808.

Weitz, R. 1993. Powerlessness, invisibility, and the lives of women with HIV disease. In *The social and behavioral aspects of AIDS: Advances in medical sociology,* vol. 3, ed. G. L. Albrecht and R. S. Zimmerman,\101–121. Greenwich, CT: JAI Press.

Whitlow, J. 1984. Jersey opens campaign to combat AIDS. *Star-Ledger* (Newark), February 9.

Whitlow, J. 1986a. Jersey now ranked third in number of AIDS cases. *Star-Ledger* (Newark), August 16.

Whitlow, J. 1986b. Jersey conducting no research on AIDS treatment. *Star-Ledger* (Newark), August 25.

Whitlow, J. 1986c. Hope and heartache go hand-in-hand for victims of AIDS. *Star-Ledger* (Newark), August 26.

Whitlow, J. 1986d. Newark protest halts AIDS nursing home. *Star-Ledger* (Newark), October 2.

Whitlow, J. 1986e. State AIDS program will provide drug treatment coupons for addicts, *Star-Ledger* (Newark), November 13.

Whitlow, J. 1987a. AIDS spreading from male drug users to women, especially minorities. *Star-Ledger* (Newark), March 1.

Whitlow, J. 1987b. Gay groups providing "straight talk" on AIDS. *Star-Ledger* (Newark), March 27.

Whitlow, J. 1987c. City, state study on Newark AIDS care facility faulted as foot-dragging. *Star-Ledger* (Newark), July 14.

Whitlow, J. 1988a. New AIDS cases in Jersey doubled during 1987. *Star-Ledger* (Newark), January 6.

Whitlow, J. 1988b. AIDS advocacy groups unite for drug research: Organizations criticize test centers, policies on improving treatment. *Star-Ledger* (Newark), August 14.

Whitlow, J. 1988c. Fighting the plague: Network of groups eases burdens of Jerseyans with AIDS. *Star-Ledger* (Newark), September 11.

Whitlow, J. 1988d. UMDNJ begins five-year study of mother-to-fetus AIDS transmission: Scientists search for treatments to prevent fatal disease in infants. *Star-Ledger* (Newark), November 15.

Whitlow, J. 1988e. Heterosexual AIDS studied in New Jersey. *Star-Ledger* (Newark), December 16.

Whitlow, J. 1991. AIDS researchers see urban Jersey developing an Africa-like epidemic. *Star-Ledger* (Newark), November 8.

Whitlow, J. 1992. AIDS testing goes mobile: Van's rounds make service accessible in low-income areas. *Star-Ledger* (Newark), August 27.

Whitlow, J. 1993. Newark failure to dole out funds costs AIDS program $5 million. *Star-Ledger* (Newark), March 18.

Whitlow, J. 1994. Against the odds: AIDS facility dedicated despite political, social obstacles. *Star-Ledger* (Newark), December 16.

Whitlow, J. 1995a. Newark seeks $8 million to fund AIDS programs in five-county area. *Star-Ledger* (Newark), February 19.

Whitlow, J. 1995b. Newark gains 6.2 million AIDS grant after resolving application errors: Aid was reduced, then cancelled due to lateness, other problems. *Star-Ledger* (Newark), March 2.

Whittaker, A. 1991. Living with HIV: Resistance by positive people. *Medical Anthropology Quarterly* 6 (4): 385–390.

Wilson, P. 1992. Health council investigates decision by Newark to rescind AIDS grants. *Star Ledger* (Newark), October 22.

Worth, D. 1986. Latina women and AIDS. *Radical America* 20 (6): 63–67.

Wu, J. A., A. S. Attele, L. Zhang, and C. S. Yuan. 2002. Anti-HIV activity of medicinal herbs: Usage and potential development. *American Journal of Chinese Medicine* 29 (1): 69–81.

Wyckoff, P. L. 1989. One baby in 22: Ominous AIDS infection rate found in Newark new-borns. *Star-Ledger* (Newark), February 14.

Wyckoff, P. L. 1993. State starts hard-hitting campaign to raise public awareness of AIDS. *Star-Ledger* (Newark), December 2.

Zippay, A., and A. Rangarajan. 2005. In their own words: WFNJ clients speak about family, work and welfare. *Work First New Jersey Evaluation*, Mathematica Policy Research, document no. PR05–26, http://www.mathematica-mpr.com/publications/PDFs/ownwords.pdf (accessed April 12, 2010).

Zsembik, B., and D. Fennell. 2005. Ethnic variation in health and the determinants of health among Latinos. *Social Science and Medicine* 61: 53–63.

INDEX

abortion, 2, 25, 74
abuse: average social/cultural capital and, 58; domestic, 59; emotional, 36, 38, 57; physical, 13, 32, 36, 38, 57; sexual, 13, 36, 37, 38, 39, 55*tab*, 56*fig*, 57, 59
ACT UP. *See* AIDS Coalition to Unleash Power
acupuncture, 66, 155, 156
ADAP. *See* AIDS Drug Assistance Program
ADAPT. *See* Association of Drug Abuse Prevention and Treatment
addiction, 93; fear of relapse into, 94; managing, 25; recovery from, 30, 37; rehabilitation programs, 48; self-curing, 32. *See also* drug use
African American(s), 2, 54; HIV/AIDS mortality rates among, 30, 70, 76; income levels, 10; racism in depictions of HIV/AIDS, 63; stereotyping of women with HIV/AIDS, 62–63
agency: development of "public voice" and, 59; on one's own behalf, 4; in structurally constrained environments, 16; structural violence and, 60; structure and, 1–20
AIDS. *See* HIV/AIDS
AIDS Clinical Trial Group 076, 63, 64, 75, 76, 77
AIDS Coalition to Unleash Power (ACT UP), 68, 78, 86
AIDS Drug Assistance Program (ADAP), 52, 106, 107
AIDS Interfaith Network, 30, 70, 76
AIDS Mastery Workshop, 76, 155
AL-721, 87
Alicia (pseudonym), 26, 54–57, 58, 94, 96, 98, 101, 103, 105, 107, 109, 133, 141, 142, 146, 148–150, 156, 159, 177–178
alliances: assistance from, 4; creation of, 29; cross-agency, 38; expertise in, 6; forming, 165*fig*; with health care professionals, 25; help in acquiring, 41; social service, 117–127, 127*fig*, 128; with social workers, 25; support group, 161*fig*
Amelia (pseudonym), 17, 19, 25, 46–48, 91, 92, 96, 100, 125–126, 148–150, 157, 175–176
anger, 27
anxiety, 156–158
ASISTENCIA (pseudonym), 119

Association of Drug Abuse Prevention and Treatment (ADAPT), 68, 69
Atripla, 187
Aviles, Armando, 79
AYUDA (pseudonym), 118, 119
AZT (azidothymidine), 43, 63, 64, 74, 76, 77, 186

Banzhaf, Marion, 77
Bardequez, Dr. Arlene, 75
Bergen, Dr. Stanley, 81
Berger, Michele, 22, 59, 96, 122, 130, 131, 134
bleach kits, 69
boarder babies, 72
Bomser, Jeffrey, 86, 87, 155
Bon Jovi, Jon, 186
Booker, Mayor Cory, 186
Boricua, 5
Bourdieu, Pierre, 16, 17, 18, 27, 164–172
Bourgois, Philippe, 16, 17
Branch, George, 80
bureaucracy: ability to manage, 28; dealing with, 6; difficulty in acclimating to demands of, 43; dominance of middle-class workers in, 6
Byrd, Frederick, 78

CAM. *See* complementary and alternative medicine
cancer, 26, 61, 62, 106, 176, 183
capital, cultural/social: ability to function and, 16; adapting to new situations and, 58; average category, 40–51, 58, 59, 137–138; bias born from, 20; broad category, 26–40, 57, 58, 60, 127; as class- and subculture-specific worldview, 17; class specificity and, 170; and clinic use, 136–142; differing treatment due to, 30, 57–58; domestic abuse and, 58; drug use and, 58; economic leverage from, 87; education and, 59; effect on health care outcomes, 20, 57–58; energy/participation level and, 147–151; experience broadening, 60; experiences leading to acquisition of, 167–168; expressed as "habitus," 17; in management of HIV/AIDS, 164–172; relation to approach to diagnosis, 146–147; risk factors for HIV/AIDS and, 24*tab*;

ABOUT THE AUTHOR

SABRINA MARIE CHASE is a medical anthropologist specializing in health disparities. She has worked with the Rutgers Center for State Health Policy and the Rutgers Institute for Health, Health Care Policy, and Aging Research. Most recently, she has been a Primary Care/Health Services Research Fellow at the Robert Wood Johnson Medical School Department of Family Medicine.

LaVergne, TN USA
11 January 2011
212079LV00001B/2/P